GASTRIC SLEEVE BARIATRIC COOKBOOK

A specific and nutritional guide on the meaning of the weight loss surgery, healing process and useful tips for a healthy diet for each stage of surgical recovery

CHAYLA HENCK

INTRODUCTION

As you probably know, there are four primary bariatric surgery procedures performed in the United States: a Roux-en-Y gastric bypass, a vertical gastrectomy sleeve (VSG), an adjustable gastric band, and a biliopancreatic bypass with a duodenal switch (BPD / DS). In 2013, the VSG has overtaken the Roux-en-Y gastric bypass as the most popular bariatric surgery in the United States.

The VSG as a unique weight-loss operation was originally the first part of a two-part bariatric surgery. Many surgeons conducted BPD / DS or gastric bypass as two consecutive procedures to reduce the risks associated with a prolonged procedure. Next, patients would have their stomach drained in an earlier, quicker, less risky operation— basically a sleeve gastrectomy.

Patients referred to the second part of the operation at a later date. Weight loss was so positive after the first phase of the treatment that some patients never returned to complete the second part of the operation. Therefore, the VSG was found to be a good weight-loss process with fewer risks than the other treatments with similar results.

Patients and providers love the gastrectomy of the sleeve. The procedure gained overwhelming popularity as a single weight-loss operation. The surgeon will remove three-fourths of the original stomach during this surgery. The banana-shaped stomach left behind is small, so it restricts the amount of food that a person can eat at any time.

During this process, no sensors are inserted. No modifications are made to any other portion of the intestinal tract of the human, which minimizes the possibility of long-term nutrient deficiencies. Throughout fact, the jacket produces great results when it comes to reducing comorbid ities, such as asthma and cardiovascular disease.

CHAPTER ONE

WHY GET SLEEVED?

Choosing sleeve gastrectomy over other forms of bariatric surgery has many benefits. Here are some of the reasons why people are choosing to get sleeved.

1. Built-in segment power.

With only 15 to 25 percent of your stomach remaining following surgery, you are constrained in the amount of food you will consume at any given moment. You can still enjoy a variety of products with a change of food flavor post-op quality, but your stomach can give strong cues to let you know when you're finished and get you to stop eating.

2. Fewer pangs of hunger.

With the removal of the majority of the stomach, the hunger hormone ghrelin has decreased. Feeling less hunger supports reduced food intake.

3. Weight loss of more than half of your total body weight.

Excessive body weight is defined as any pound above your calculated ideal body weight for your height. Research reported by the American Society for Metabolic and Bariatric Surgery Integrated

Health Nutritional Guidelines for Surgical Weight Loss Patients shows that people are able to maintain a weight loss of more than 55% of their excess body weight five years or more after surgery. For an individual who is 150 pounds in excess of their ideal weight, this means keeping at least 80 pounds off for the long term.

4. Eat candy with no wasting condition.
Many people have a hard time talking about giving up birthday cake or special-occasion ice cream for the rest of their lives following weight-loss surgery. Dumping syndrome is a disorder that may arise in individuals who have had gastric bypass or BPD / DS surgery after eating foods high in sugar and, in some instances, having too many carbs at one time.

Symptoms occur immediately after the meal in question and include a mixture of feeling nervous, light-headed, sweating or dizzy; elevated pulse rate; reduced blood sugar levels (reactive hypoglycemia); abdominal cramping; and diarrhea. Although large quantities of sweets may still cause dumping-like symptoms after VSG, it is very rare and not as severe as after weight-loss surgery, which involves the modification of the small intestine.

LESS TIME IN THE OPERATING ROOM

Any operation performed under general anesthesia involves risks and the potential for complications. These risks may multiply with the amount of time the operation takes to complete. Although the VSG is a longer treatment than the elastic brace, it is a quicker and easier method than the gastric bypass and the BPD / DS.

IF YOU CONSIDERING GASTRIC BYPASS

The main difference between the gastric bypass and the VSG is the second step of the gastric bypass process requiring the rerouting of the narrow intestinal tract. During the gastric bypass operation, a narrow cavity is developed from the wider stomach and part of the small intestinal tract is separated and attached to the new stomach.

To this end, the end side of the stomach and the upper part of the small intestinal tract are "deviated" during the digestion of food.

Similar to sleeve gastrectomy, gastric bypass produces slightly higher weight loss in the short term and slightly higher levels of type 2 diabetes resolution.

Dump syndrome may occur after gastric bypass when patients eat sweets. Dumping syndrome is often a good barrier to eating sweets for people struggling to minimize the calorie intake of sugary foods.

Another difference between gastric bypass and sleeve gastrectomy is that the gastric bypass immediately resolves any symptoms of gastroesophageal reflux disease or GERD after surgery. Following VSG, reflux can potentially get worse directly following surgery, but often improves with time. It is very important to discuss in depth the essence of your own behaviors and health history with your physician and medical team to decide which operation is better for you in the long term.

The recommendations for gastric bypass and VSG are very close when it comes to post-op care. You can still plan all the recipes for this book without having to worry over texture or section if you decide for a bypass.

Beginning with Nutrition A full team of medical professionals, comprising, at a minimum, a physician, a registered dietitian and a counselor, will help you better appreciate the operation as well as how to plan for it emotionally, psychologically and nutritionally.

But in the days, weeks, and years following surgery, success will depend on your ability to start with food in a real and lasting way. Part of this reset includes self-education in diet, and the other part requires self-management, which can be the hardest part of it.

CHALLENGES PEOPLE FACE AFTER SURGERY.

Embracing Food without Anxiety Through bariatric surgery, you decide to learn how to eat all over again. Beginning with only drinks, you can gradually move on to a balanced diet of almost all the food you might consume before surgery. You might be afraid to know just what's safe to eat, and you don't really want to eat again because of this anxiety.

In addition, you may be afraid of falling into old eating habits and losing the benefits of surgery. For accept food without doubt, concentrate on what you can consume instead of what you can't eat.

Stick to the basic principles of bariatric diet and choose to eat the food you know you can eat. It's going to take months for you to have complete confidence in your dos and don't have a bariatric diet, so give yourself time and don't try right away. If you stick to the rules for the first few weeks, you're not going to get sick. Time. Period. After that, listen to your body's messages.

Be patient and make every effort to stop eating at the first hint of fullness. Tap into your body's natural cues and stop taking another bite until you feel full. You don't have to live in fear; your body is going to tell you when to stop.

Come on to yourself. It's really different this time. You might be afraid to go back to the "old you" just like you used to die in the past. But now you've got the help of this beneficial surgery, which gives you a great start to your head. Now you're not just starting a diet, you're starting a whole lifestyle change: a permanent lifestyle change without turning back.

Recognize that support is of paramount importance. At least focus on your medical professionals, and hopefully at least a few associates, families, or colleagues. Turn to the people you trust to be encouraged when you feel scared. If you feel like you don't have anyone to support you, check again.

There's someone— a bariatric support group, a health coach, a psychologist, a pastor, a colleague. Talk with the one who can really motivate you through the bumps on the bridge. You become mentally and physically impaired from living in fear. Be assured that you can be effective in the post-op process and be aware of the choices you make every day.

CONTROLLING URGES
We've all got urges. Whether it's an impulse purchase at the mall, a second dessert help, or a wasteful day watching Netflix and a lack of workout— there are plenty of opportunities to give in and fall off your healthy lifestyle. The control of urges involves two parts.

1. Improve your mindfulness. Being mindful of your emotions, desires, and behavior in the present moment will help to curb your urges.

2. Don't give in to your cravings. For some individuals, giving in to temptation involves flipping a key, putting it back into an "on" role that might have been blocked. How many times does eating a chip turn into half a bag, drinking a glass of wine into half a bottle, or eating an Oreo turn into a whole sleeve? For many bariatric patients, giving in to desires, compulsions, or impulses can contribute to binge-type behavior.

Practice awareness and remind yourself if this is what the body actually needs at the moment. Sometimes the reaction is "yeah," that's just what you need. Yet stop and ask again before giving in to a slight impulse, as it often adds to a domino effect in self-harming habits.

DEMONSTRATING SELF-COMPASSION
What we act about ourselves and what we handle ourselves for good and bad attitudes directly affects our satisfaction. It can also affect our ability to keep up with long-term behavioral changes following surgery. The doctor describes self-compassion as three parts— self-kindness, empathy, and common humanity.

During treatment, both patients make mistakes. It's whether we react with self-compassion or self-criticism that defines how strong we are after a time of slipping back into old habits. We are all individual, and we have our own imperfections. Take advantage of your good qualities and accept your challenges, too.

Seek to use your talents to solve challenges in other fields. Self-denigration is only going to move you farther further from your ambitions. When you've got a couple of bad days, realize that your subconscious might have needed a break.

Try to move forward without focusing too much on past mistakes, and look forward to your continued success.

APPRECIATING NATURAL SWEETNESS

We live in a culture where our threshold for sweetness is growing higher and higher. Desserts are growing increasingly natural and soft beverages are becoming sweeter. Changing the habit of eating candy can be especially difficult for anyone trying to lose weight because sugar is addictive.

Eating sugary snacks turns your brain's pleasure centers light, causing you want to go out for more. If this is something you've been struggling with, bariatric surgery gives you the chance to press the reset button. You're going to get a redo on your food preferences and an opportunity to get some major help in pushing old habits to the edge.

Focus on eating naturally sweet food to balance your need to satisfy all taste buds. Include grains such as barley or quinoa, which have a sweet and nutty flavor and are still packed with plenty of nutrients. Instead of sugary desserts, top off your meal with something naturally sweet like fresh berries or fresh citrus fruits

Even using 100% cocoa powder in protein shakes or other baked goods, you can reduce your chocolate cravings without extra sugar and fat from typical milk chocolate candies. Appreciating the natural sweetness of food will help to put down the sugar addiction!

MANAGING WEIGHT — Management EXPECTATIONS

Weight loss is not a perfect science. Even in a controlled weight-loss study, there is still some variation in the weight loss of individuals. It's hard to send you a 110 percent commitment, and the outcomes aren't what you expect. To order to manage the post-op weight loss goals, don't put undue strain on yourself to lose weight more rapidly than is practical. Okay, learn yourself. Others may lose weight faster or slower than you do.

The causes that lead in weight loss are multifaceted and some are out of your influence. Did you know that weight loss might even affect the amount of sleep you get? In addition to food intake, exercise, muscle mass, stress, starting body weight, height, gender, age, and even more factors all play a part in the amount of weight you lose. Be vigilant, and polite, and don't equate yourself with others.

Your weight-loss path is unique; it's all right and you're going to be disappointed at times. Just know that you will achieve long-term success with continued hard work.

ENJOYING FOOD AGAIN
During the first few days of post-op, when you consume mostly liquids, it's hard to imagine that you'll ever find pleasure in eating food again.

Initially, it can be a chore, something done out of necessity.

Questions can begin to flutter: can I look forward to eating again? Will I ever be able to eat the food I used to love?
Keep in mind that right after surgery, your body undergoes rapid physical and hormonal changes— all of which suppress your urge to eat and the amount you can eat.

Most of your initial rapid weight loss is the result of a combination of these changes. Be patient with me. When time progresses, you will be comfortable and able to eat a slightly larger amount of food and accept a wider variety of foods.

I know this may sound untrue, but some people who really enjoyed pizza and ice cream before surgery may no longer want to consume certain kinds of food. When you move on to a diet full of nutritious foods and leaving aside high-calorie foods, you will notice that your body is more ready for healthier foods. And this is the best time to try some of your favorite old recipes— with a safer twist.

Food is food for your body; it's a must to feed every single day. Yet mealtime is so much more than what we place in our mouths. With a little preparation, flexibility, and willingness to experiment, it's really possible to enjoy nutritious food after surgery.

FREQUENTLY ASKED QUESTIONS

After surgery, stay connected to your bariatric medical team and support group so that you can easily get answers to your questions and concerns from a reliable source— and receive support and encouragement. Here are a few questions that I have frequently been asked.

Taking a walk down the nutrition and vitamin row in your grocery store may be daunting. There are hundreds of products on the market, each of which promises to be different than the next. You want to set a strong diet plan because you're not going to drink protein shakes for the rest of your life. Protein shakes and powders should be a bridge for the first few days and weeks to allow you to eat whole foods. In comparison, protein powders can be used to help you easily take in a rich source of high-quality protein with very few calories. Here are my guidelines for bariatric-friendly protein powder.

Choose the protein whey isolate. It's easier for your body to absorb, and it's dense in essential amino acids. Other high quality sources include soya protein (vegan) isolates or egg white powders.
Use some unflavored protein powder. We are low in calories and the cleanest since they are safe from artificial ingredients.

Use sugar-free with flavored protein powders
Okay, look for completely sugar-free varieties that are sweetened with stevia, sucralose (Splenda) or other sugar substitutes. There are hundreds of taste choices from coffee to pecan oil, so you'll be pleased with very few calories. Sugar substitutes are FDA-approved, calorie-free, and healthy to use after surgery.

Be vigilant of sugar alcohols (erythritol, mannitol, xylitol, and sorbitol) because they add calories and may induce unwanted gastrointestinal side effects. Find the sample sizes you need to try before your surgery. Search for free or discounted products on the manufacturer's website. This way, you'll realize what you like and what you don't have in order for the first few days of post-op.

Get something quick and easy, such as low-fat cottage cheese or Greek yogurt, hard-boiled eggs, nitrate-free turkey or chicken lunch meat or low-fat cheese. Milk or protein shake may also fulfill the protein target. The key is to focus on hitting your protein target at least 80% of the time. Begin the next day with a high-protein breakfast to make up for what you might have lost the day before.

It seems impossible that eating straight protein foods for weeks and months to come could be considered a healthy lifestyle, but it's only temporary. The multivitamin should mask what you're going to lose of nutrients during this process. Work on making it a priority to consume fruit and vegetables as the first items you choose once you're able to spread past proteins.

Various types of fruit and vegetables throughout the week since it's hard to eat a few portions in a single day. There are hundreds of recipes in this book that give tips on how to slip fruit and vegetables right into your main protein dishes. Work your way up to five servings of fruit and vegetables a day in the long run.

There are two specific reasons why people do not eat doughy bread products and pasta following surgery. The first is that the current stomach is not well handled. The sleeve has a hard time digesting these foods in the first few months. If you eat them, you may feel overly full quickly and then hungry shortly after, or you may feel bloated, and/or you may feel that something is stuck in your small stomach.

Such symptoms usually arise after the first few months, but some people experience pain from consuming such types of foods over the longer term. The second reason people restrict carbohydrate intake is to rely more on consuming protein foods for fullness and fruits and vegetables that are low in calories. It's not bad to eat bread and pasta following surgery if you can handle it — it should be mild, concentrating first on nutrition, then fruits, then carbs.

It's ideal to enlist the support of loved ones, partners, family, and friends before surgery, but you can't always wait to change your lifestyle until everyone you know is equally ready. Here are a few tips to stay on track when the rest of the household might be more resistant.

Hold the most enticing remedies out of the pantry. Allow only the convenient rewards that you can avoid. Oreos may be your greatest weakness, but the rest of the household couldn't care less if the cookies were Chips Ahoy or Nutter Butters. Don't buy Oreos, but let family favorites do not tempt you.

Figure out the source. Whether it's heading out for a stroll, going to bed early, getting lost in a good book, or texting a friend — find an outlet for pain, fear, or depression that's not eating. Make sure you have an alternate option for yourself when your name is called by the potato chips.

Have simple meals on hand for yourself and the rest of your family. Make every effort to stop becoming a short-term post-op chef. Have some food on hand so there's always something safe, simple, and easy going around. When appropriate, consider foods that can be quickly changed to suit your needs and the taste preferences of others.

Tell about what you need. Not everyone in the family will appreciate the wishes while you adopt a bariatric diet. Practice good communication and make sure you know what you need for support.

You can't assume that other people know what your objectives are and what you need to do.

Weight-loss surgery is a procedure on your chest, but it does not alter the pre-operative eating habits in your head. With that in mind, I strongly suggest that patients establish as many healthy and positive eating patterns ahead of time with a post-op diet in mind. Keeping the patterns in order before treatment will make things a lot easier when you're healing.

It's overwhelming to ask yourself how to count protein grams, give up fast food, stop drinking liquids with food, and start taking multivitamin supplements all at once. Whether or not the surgical center needs you to adopt a pre-operative regimen of some kind is independent of your preference to develop as many post-op routines as practicable in advance of time.

Most bariatric surgery plans and/or insurance companies include some kind of pre-operative weight loss, high-protein diet, or liquid diet within days, weeks, and sometimes months before surgery. Losing weight in the last week or two before surgery, particularly through a low-carbohydrate or liquid diet, can help to reduce the size of the liver and lower abdominal fat, making surgery simpler for the surgeon and healthier for you.

Just Keep Trying When you wake up from bariatric surgery, your entire lifestyle will only change if you choose to make it different. Surgery doesn't prohibit you from eating fast food. Surgery doesn't allow you get out of the sofa. Surgery doesn't stop you from having a bag of potato chips every dinner.

Modifying a century of behaviors to meet your weight loss goals can be difficult. Although you're going to face hurdles and challenges, just keep trying. Babies don't learn how to run before they can walk about. So just do these small things. You may only be able to walk for 10 minutes without getting exhausted, but 10 minutes is a start.

You may not be able to give up candy entirely, but you can mix in smaller portions. You may not be able to give up fast food, but you can get a burger without a side of the fries. Small steps are making a difference. Set realistic, attainable goals for yourself. You're going to have weeks when the pounds fall off in double digits, and weeks when you don't seem to be making the scale budge. Don't give it up. Don't lose your hope. Just keep on trying. Keep a food log for a couple of days. Try a new kind of fitness class. Go to bed 30 minutes earlier to get some extra sleep. Schedule a follow-up to your bariatric medical team. Just keep on trying.

ALCOHOL AFTER VSG

When you had a few alcoholic beverages before bariatric surgery, and you're curious if this is something you should proceed with after treatment, you should have a good understanding of how the operation will impact the absorption of alcohol. There is an enzyme in the stomach that helps partially digest alcohol. Since most of the stomach is eliminated during VSG, the capacity to break down alcohol will be significantly altered.

As a consequence, even a tiny amount of alcohol consumption is highly intoxicating. The smaller body size and limited food intake will also lead to alcohol intoxication and dehydration. Moreover, alcohol is extremely dense in calories. Bariatric surgery does not restrict liquid calories, and alcohol calories can add up very quickly.

Weddings, family gatherings, parties— alcohol can be a major part of socializing, but for many post-op patients, alcohol intake can be a replacement for food as an outlet from pain. According to the Obesity Action Coalition, the likelihood of relapse following bariatric surgery is increased due to something called a transition of addiction. People trade drug consumption as an escape for pain, sadness, or anxiety. And think twice before drinking champagne following surgery — think about making yourself a designated driver and go for non-alcoholic drinks instead.

When drinking is a problem for you or your loved one, realize that your bariatric medical team is there to serve you; assistance is waiting for you. Alcoholism is not supposed to be kept hidden, and you are not alone. You can also find information about Alcoholics Anonymous in the Resources section of this report. Alcoholics Anonymous can help you determine if you have a problem with the transfer of addiction and help you fight it.

CHAPTER TWO
BREAKFAST

SOUTHWESTERN SCRAMBLED EGG BURRITOS

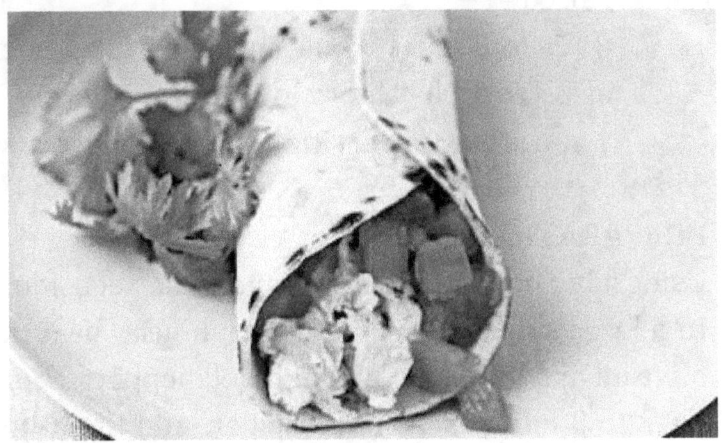

PREP TIME: 10 MINUTES
COOK TIME: 10 MINUTES
TOTAL TIME: 20 MINUTES
SERVINGS: 8

These breakfast burritos have the ingredients you crave but without all the added sodium and fat. Make them freeze and then toss one in the microwave for a hot breakfast in minutes.

INGREDIENTS

- 12 eggs
- ¼ cup low-fat milk

- 1 teaspoon extra-virgin olive oil
- ½ onion, chopped
- 1 red bell pepper, diced
- 1 green bell pepper, diced
- 1 (15-ounce) can black beans, drained and rinsed
- 8 (7- to 8-inch) whole-wheat tortillas, such as La Tortilla Factory low-carb tortillas
- 1 cup salsa, for serving

PREPARATIONS

Using a big bowl stir the eggs and milk. Set aside.
In a large skillet over medium-high heat, heat the olive oil and add the onion and bell peppers. Sauté for 2 to 3 minutes, or until tender. Add the beans and stir to combine.
Add the egg mixture. Minimize heat and mix while constantly with a rubber spatula for 5 minutes, until the eggs are fluffy and cooked through.

Divide the scrambled egg mixture among the tortillas. Fold over the bottom end of the tortilla, fold in the sides, and roll tightly to close.
Serve immediately with the salsa, or place each burrito in a zip-top bag and refrigerate for up to 1 week. To eat, reheat each burrito in the

microwave for 60 to 90 seconds. These will also keep well in the freezer for up to 1 month.

Serving tip: To get more vegetables into your breakfast, buy a bag of frozen California-blend mixed vegetables. Heat some in a skillet with extra-virgin olive oil, add eggs, and—voilà!—a quick veggie-packed egg burrito.

NUTRITIONAL VALUE
Per Serving (1 burrito): Calories: 250; Total fat: 10g; Protein: 19g; Carbs: 28g; Fiber: 13g; Sugar: 1g; Sodium: 546mg

SMOOTHIE BOWL WITH GREEK YOGURT AND FRESH BERRIES

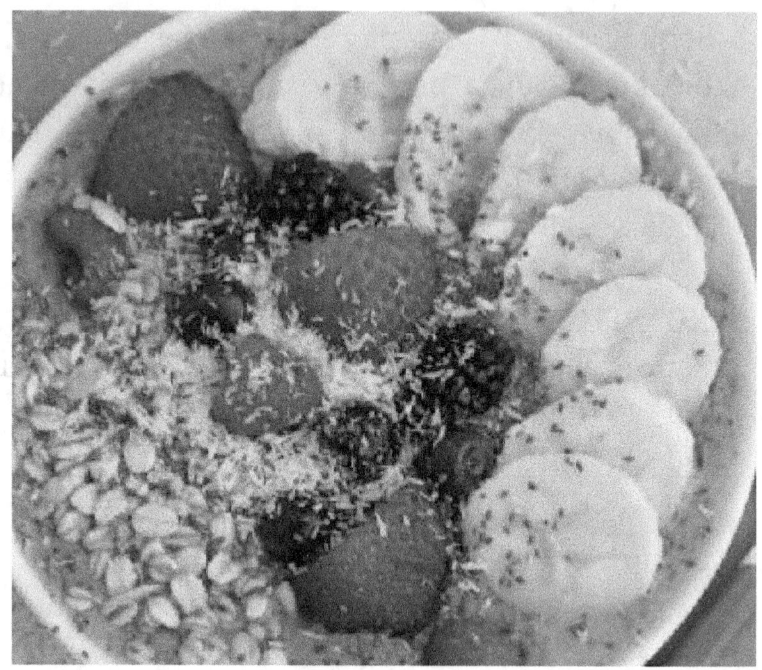

PREP TIME: 5 MINUTES
COOK TIME: 5 MINUTES
TOTAL TIME: 10 MINUTES
SERVINGS: 1

The appearance of our food and where we eat our meals can strongly affect our feelings of satiety after eating. In fact, after surgery, whether you're eating in a high-stress environment or having a relaxing candlelit dinner can influence whether a food makes you sick. Instead of slamming a protein shake for your next breakfast on the way out the door, try sitting down to enjoy this refreshing smoothie bowl. It is just as appealing to the eye as the stomach. Slow down and savor every bite of this smoothie you can eat with a spoon!

INGREDIENTS

- ¾ cup unsweetened vanilla almond milk or low-fat milk
- ¼ cup low-fat plain Greek yogurt
- ⅓ cup (1 handful) fresh spinach
- ½ scoop (⅛ cup) plain or vanilla protein powder
- ¼ cup frozen mixed berries
- ¼ cup fresh raspberries
- ¼ cup fresh blueberries
- 1 tablespoon sliced, slivered almonds
- 1 teaspoon chia seeds

PREPARATION

In a blender, combine the milk, yogurt, spinach, protein powder, and frozen berries. For 4 minutes blend, until the powder is well dissolved and no longer visible.

Pour the smoothie into small bowl.

Decorate the smoothie with the fresh raspberries, blueberries, almonds, and chia seeds.

Serve with a spoon and enjoy!

Serving tip: You can make this smoothie bowl with a variety of other fruits and toppings to change it up. Try a mango-pineapple version. Top with unsweetened, flaked coconut and use coconut milk in the smoothie base for a more tropical vibe.

NUTRITIONAL VALUE

Per Serving (1 bowl): Calories: 255; Total fat: 10 g; Protein: 20g; Carbs: 21g; Fiber: 8g; Sugar: 10g; Sodium: 262mg

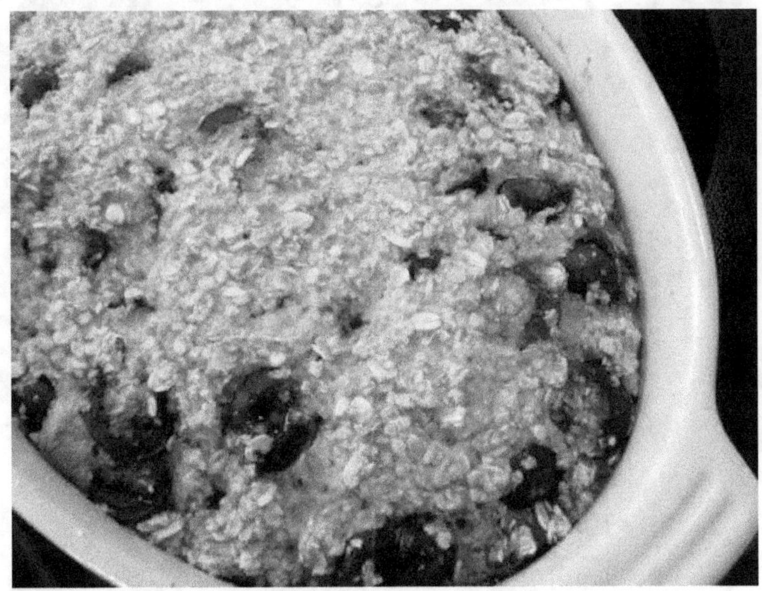

PREP TIME: 10 MINUTES
COOK TIME: 45 MINUTES
TOTAL TIME: 55 MINUTES
SERVINGS: 6

Look no farther than this baked oatmeal recipe to replace your run-of-the-mill coffee shop pastry— the ones that are high in sugar, high in fat, and high in calories. The sweet flavor and hearty ingredients of this baked oatmeal will leave you feeling warm and satisfied on any cold winter morning. Bake for Sunday breakfast and eat leftovers throughout the week.

INGREDIENTS

- Nonstick cooking spray
- 1 cup old-fashioned oats
- ½ teaspoon ground cinnamon
- ¾ teaspoon baking powder
- 1 tablespoon ground flaxseed
- 3 eggs
- 1 cup low-fat milk
- ½ cup low-fat plain Greek yogurt
- 1 teaspoon vanilla extract
- 1 teaspoon liquid stevia (optional; to improve sweetness)
- 1 cup fresh pitted cherries
- 1 apple, peeled, cored and chopped

PREPARATION

Preheat the oven to 375°F. Lightly coat an 8-by-8-inch baking dish with the cooking spray.

Mix together the oats, cinnamon, baking powder, and flaxseed in a medium bowl. In a separate large bowl, gently whisk the eggs, milk, yogurt, vanilla, and stevia (if using).

Combine the dry ingredients and mix to combine. Gently fold in the cherries and apples.

Bake for 45 minutes or until the edges start to pull away from the side of the pan and the oatmeal gently bounces back when touched.
Divide leftover oatmeal into airtight glass containers. Refrigerate for up to 1 week for quick and easy breakfast, or freeze.

Serving tip: Experiment with the fixings in your baked oatmeal. I like to make my recipes seasonal. Replace the yogurt with pumpkin puree to add a hint of fall. Try using unsweetened dried cranberries instead of cherries for a holiday twist. Swap out apples and cherries for 2 cups fresh berries in spring for a very berry oatmeal! For the creamiest consistency, I recommend topping with a ¼ cup low-fat milk at serving time.

NUTRITIONAL VALUE
Per Serving (½ cup): Calories: 149; Total fat: 4g; Protein: 8g; Carbs: 21g; Fiber: 4g; Sugar: 9g; Sodium: 71 mg

HIGH-PROTEIN PANCAKES
PREP TIME: 5 MINUTES
COOK TIME: 5 MINUTES
TOTAL TIME: 10 MINUTES

SERVINGS: 4

Try these high-protein pancakes this weekend. Made with simple ingredients already in your pantry and refrigerator, these hotcakes are sure to be a crowd pleaser.

INGREDIENTS

- 3 eggs
- 1 cup low-fat cottage cheese
- ⅓ cup whole-wheat pastry flour
- 1½ tablespoons coconut oil, melted
- Nonstick cooking spray

PREPARATIONS

In large bowl, lightly whisk the eggs.

Whisk in the cottage cheese, flour, and coconut oil just until combined.

Heat a large skillet or griddle over medium heat, and lightly coat with the cooking spray.

Using a measuring cup, pour ⅓ cup of batter into the skillet for each pancake, Boil   for 3 minutes and till bubbles appear across the surface of each pancake

Flip over the pancakes and cook for 1 to 2 minutes on the other side, or until golden brown.

Serve immediately.

Serving tip: Top these pancakes with fresh berries and plain yogurt, unsweetened applesauce, or sugar-free syrup. You can even try them with natural peanut butter and bananas on a general diet.

NUTRITIONAL VALUE
Per Serving (1 pancake): Calories: 182; Total fat: 10g; Protein: 12g; Carbs: 10g; Fiber: 3g; Sugar: 1g; Sodium: 68mg

PUMPKIN MUFFINS WITH WALNUTS AND ZUCCHINI

PREP TIME: 10 MINUTES
COOK TIME: 25 MINUTES
TOTAL TIME: 35 MINUTES
SERVINGS: 4

Most muffins you pick up at your local bakery are packed with loads of sugar, white flour, and plenty of fat. Luckily, it's easy to make your own soft and delicious muffins at home with a few healthy twists. These muffins stay light and moist because they are made with shredded zucchini and pureed pumpkin.

INGREDIENTS
- Nonstick cooking spray or baking liners
- 2 cups old-fashioned oats
- 1¾ cups whole-wheat pastry flour

- ¼ cup ground flaxseed
- 2 tablespoons baking powder
- 1 teaspoon baking soda
- 1 teaspoon ground cinnamon
- ¼ teaspoon ground nutmeg
- ¼ teaspoon ground ginger
- ¼ teaspoon ground allspice
- 2 cups shredded zucchini
- 1 cup canned pumpkin or fresh pumpkin puree
- 1 cup low-fat milk
- 4 eggs, lightly beaten
- ¼ cup unsweetened applesauce
- 1 teaspoon liquid stevia
- ½ cup chopped walnuts

PREPARATIONS

Preheat the oven to 375°F. Prepare two muffin tins by coating the cups with the cooking spray, or use baking liners.

In large bowl, mix together the oats, flour, flaxseed, baking powder, baking soda, cinnamon, nutmeg, ginger, and allspice.

In a separate medium bowl mix together the zucchini, pumpkin, milk, eggs, applesauce, and stevia

Add the wet ingredients to the dry and stir to combine. Gently stir in the walnuts.

Fill the cups of the muffin tins about half full with the batter.

Bake until the muffins are done, when a toothpick inserted in the center comes out clean, about 25 minutes.

Let the muffins cool for 5 minutes before removing them from the tins. Place on a baking rack to finish cooling.

Wrap leftover muffins in plastic wrap and freeze. Reheat frozen muffins in the microwave for about 20 seconds.

Ingredient tip: Put the shredded zucchini in a colander in the sink and press it with the back of a spoon to drain the moisture; pat dry with paper towels before adding to the bowl.

Did You Know? Flaxseed is rich in omega-3s. Omega-3 fats have anti-inflammatory effects in the body and may help promote a healthy brain and healthy heart. Ground flaxseed is also a great source of fiber. It can be mixed into smoothies, cereal, or yogurt. It can also be easily added to baked goods. Swap out ¼ cup of flour for ¼ cup of ground flaxseed in any baking recipe to get more of this nutrient-packed seed into your diet!

NUTRITIONAL VALUE

Per Serving (1 muffin): Calories: 128; Total fat: 5g; Protein: 5g; Carbs: 18g; Fiber: 3g; Sugar: 1g; Sodium: 86mg

HARD-BOILED EGGS AND AVOCADO ON TOAST

PREP TIME: 10 MINUTES

COOK TIME: 10 MINUTES

TOTAL TIME: 20 MINUTES

SERVINGS: 4

A diet staple after a sleeve gastrectomy, eggs are packed with protein, vitamins, and minerals. Eggs are rich in choline, which is essential for brain and liver function. Choose organic free-range eggs when possible, as their yolks contain more heart-healthy omega-3 fats than conventional versions. Hard-boil a dozen eggs at a time and keep them on hand to eat throughout the week.

INGREDIENTS

- 4 eggs

- 4 slices sprouted whole-wheat bread, such as Angelic Bakehouse Sprouted Grain
- 1 medium avocado
- 1 teaspoon hot sauce
- Freshly ground black pepper
-

PREPARATIONS

Using a pot fill it up and rapid boil over high heat.

Carefully add the eggs to the boiling water using a spoon, and set a timer for 10 minutes.

Immediately transfer the eggs from the boiling water to a strainer, and run cold water over the eggs to stop the cooking process.

Once the eggs are cool enough to handle, peel them and slice lengthwise into fourths.

Toast the bread.

While the bread toasts, mash the avocado with a fork in a small bowl and mix in the hot sauce.

Spread the avocado mash evenly across each toast. Top each toast slice with 4 egg slices and season with the black pepper.

Ingredient tip: Avocado is rich in healthy fat, but also loaded with calories, so portion control is key. Store the pit with any unused portion of avocado, squeeze a teaspoon of lemon juice over the leftovers, and place in an airtight container or wrap in plastic wrap to prevent browning.

NUTRITIONAL VALUE

Per Serving (1 toast): Calories: 191; Total fat: 10g; Protein: 10g; Carbs: 15g; Fiber: 5g; Sugar: 1g; Sodium: 214mg

CHAPTER THREE
VEGETARIAN DINNERS

MEXICAN STUFFED SUMMER SQUASH

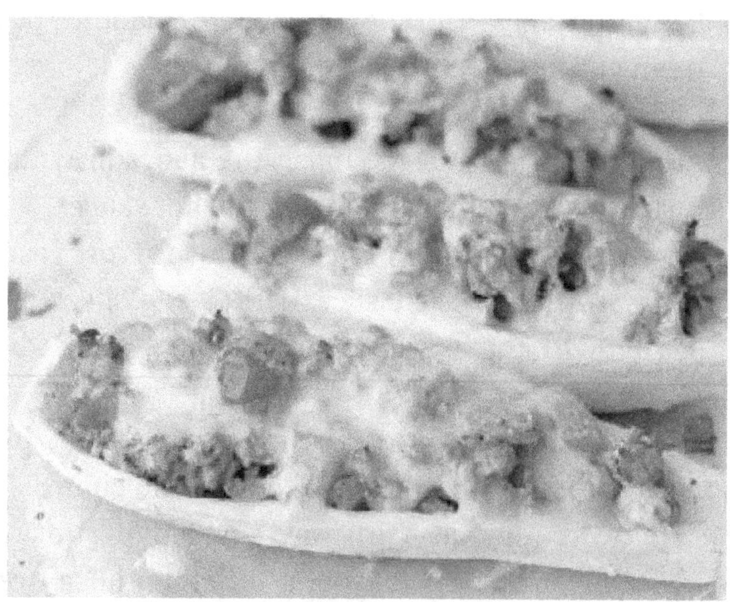

PREP TIME: 5 MINUTES

COOK TIME: 33 MINUTES
TOTAL TIME: 38 MINUTES
SERVINGS: 2
Here is a great low-carb dish that will satisfy your cravings and use some of summer's most plentiful vegetables. It's easy enough to double or triple to make for a family or for you to eat throughout the week.

INGREDIENTS

- Nonstick cooking spray
- 1 yellow summer squash
- ½ cup Refried Black Beans or canned fat-free refried pinto beans with 1 teaspoon taco seasoning mixed in (for flavor)
- ½ cup cooked quinoa
- ¼ cup shredded Colby Jack cheese
- 1 small tomato, diced
- 2 tablespoons sliced black olives
- 2 scallions, chopped, for garnish

PREPARATIONS

Preheat the oven to 400°F. Coat an 8-by-8-inch baking dish with the cooking spray.

Cut the ends off of the summer squash and discard. Cut lengthwise, then use a spoon to remove and discard the seeds. Place the squash halves cut-side down in the baking dish. Gently poke a couple of holes in the squash to vent. Add 1 tablespoon of water to the dish. Microwave for about 3 minutes or until slightly tender. Discard any leftover water.

When cool enough to handle, turn the squash so they are skin-side down and spaced evenly apart in the dish.

Layer ¼ cup of the beans in each squash, then ¼ cup of the quinoa, Top the whole thing with the Colby Jack cheese. Cover with aluminum foil and bake for 25 minutes. Remove the foil and bake for 5 minutes more, or until the cheese is bubbly and the squash is tender.

Garnish each squash with the tomatoes, olives, and scallions just before serving.

Serving tip: Get creative with extras. Brown ground turkey or a soy-based meat substitute in taco seasoning and add on top of the beans. Sauté bell peppers and onions to layer on or serve with avocado and cilantro

NUTRITIONAL VALUE

Per Serving (1 squash half): Calories: 190; Total fat: 8 g; Protein: 9g; Carbs: 21g; Fiber: 4g; Sugar: 3g; Sodium: 40mg

ROASTED VEGETABLE QUINOA SALAD WITH CHICKPEAS

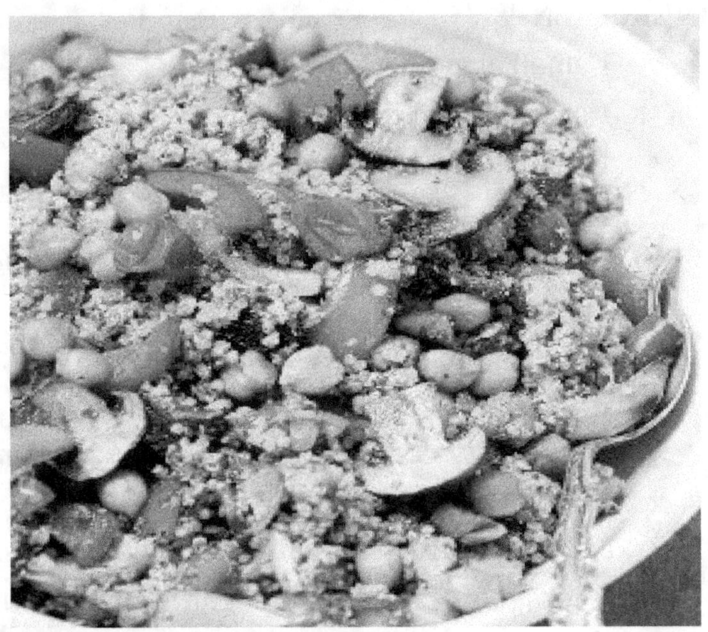

PREP TIME: 15 MINUTES
COOK TIME: 30 MINUTES
TOTAL TIME: 45 MINUTES
SERVINGS: 6

Many people find that their sleeve tolerates cooked vegetables better than raw vegetables in the initial months post-op. This quinoa salad is an excellent alternative to traditional lettuce salads. It contains a variety of vegetarian protein sources—quinoa and chickpeas—and it's loaded with vegetables that have been roasted to bring out their natural rich flavors.

INGREDIENTS

- 1 small eggplant, diced
- 1 small zucchini, diced
- 1 small yellow summer squash, diced
- ½ cup grape tomatoes, halved
- 1 (15-ounce) can chickpeas, drained and rinsed
- 3 tablespoons extra-virgin olive oil, divided
- ⅓ cup packaged quinoa
- 1 cup low-sodium vegetable or chicken broth
- 2 tablespoons freshly squeezed lemon juice
- 1 teaspoon minced fresh garlic or 1 garlic clove, minced
- 1 tablespoon dried basil
- 1 teaspoon dried oregano

PREPARATIONS

Preheat the oven to 425°F. Line a 9-by-13-inch baking sheet with parchment paper.

Spread the eggplant, zucchini, yellow squash, tomatoes, and chickpeas across the baking sheet and toss them with 1 tablespoon of olive oil.

Bake for 30 minutes, stirring once halfway through. The finished vegetables should be tender and the tomatoes should be juicy. The chickpeas will be firm and crispy.

While the vegetables and chickpeas are roasting, place the quinoa and broth in a small saucepan over medium-high heat. Cover and bring to a boil. Minimize heat and boil for about 15 minutes, or until all liquid has absorbed. Remove the pan from the heat and fluff the quinoa with a fork. (Otherwise, make the quinoa according to the package instructions.)

In a small dish, whisk together the lemon juice, garlic, and remaining 2 tablespoons of olive oil. Mix in the basil and oregano.

Using a big bowl mix the quinoa, roasted vegetables with chickpeas, and dressing. Gently stir to combine. Serve and enjoy!

Serving tip: To increase the protein in this dish, you can add lean grilled chicken breast or serve with a piece of baked fish. You can always top with a dollop of low-fat plain Greek yogurt.

NUTRITIONAL VALUE

Per Serving (½ cup): Calories: 200; Total fat: 9g; Protein: 7g; Carbs: 27g; Fiber: 8g; Sugar: 4g; Sodium: 160mg

RED LENTIL SOUP WITH KALE

PREP TIME: 10 MINUTES
COOK TIME: 45 MINUTES
TOTAL TIME: 55 MINUTES
SERVINGS: 6

Eating vegetarian can be just as filling as eating a diet high in animal protein when you choose the right foods. Warm up with this hearty lentil soup—loaded with filling fiber and flavorful herbs and seasonings. Keep a bag of lentils on hand so you can whip up this hearty soup on the next cold winter night.

INGREDIENTS

- 1 tablespoon extra-virgin olive oil
- 1 cup chopped onion
- ½ cup carrots, cut into ½-inch chunks
- ½ cup celery, cut into ¼-inch chunks
- 1 teaspoon minced garlic
- 1 cup red lentils
- 1 teaspoon dried thyme
- 1 teaspoon ground cumin

- 2 cups low-sodium vegetable broth
- 2 cups water
- 2 large stalks kale, stemmed, with leaves chopped (about 2 cups)
- 1 bay leaf
- 2 tablespoons freshly squeezed lemon juice
- Low-fat plain Greek yogurt (optional)

PREPARATIONS

In a large stock pot over medium heat, heat the olive oil. Add the onion, carrots, celery, and garlic, and sauté until tender, 5 to 7 minutes.

Add the lentils, thyme, and cumin. Mix well and stir for 1 to 2 minutes, until all the ingredients are coated well with the seasonings.

Add the broth and water to the pot. Bring to a simmer, add the kale, and stir well. Add the bay leaf, then cover the pot and simmer for 30 to 35 minutes.

Remove the pot from the heat. Remove and discard the bay leaf. Stir in the lemon juice. Use an immersion blender to puree the soup to your desired consistency. Alternatively, let the soup cool for 10 minutes before pureeing it in batches in a blender.

Garnish each bowl of soup with a dollop of the Greek yogurt (if using) and serve.

Post-op tip: If you're cooking this during the post-op pureed stage, add 1 to 2 tablespoons of egg white powder or unflavored protein powder after cooking to increase the protein content.

NUTRITIONAL VALUE

Per Serving (1 cup): Calories: 170; Total fat: 3g; Protein: 13g; Carbs: 24g; Fiber: 3g; Sugar: 4g; Sodium: 59mg

CHEESY BROCCOLI SOUP

PREP TIME: 10 MINUTES
COOK TIME: 20 MINUTES
TOTAL TIME: 30 MINUTES
SERVINGS: 2

Who doesn't love Panera Bread's Broccoli Cheddar soup? It's so rich, creamy, and satisfying. Knowing these are the types of meals my patients craved in the months after bariatric surgery, I set out to create my own version that offers all the flavor and texture of the soup with far fewer calories and less fat. I hope this recipe will have your taste buds and your family fooled!

INGREDIENTS

- 1 tablespoon extra-virgin olive oil
- 1 medium onion, chopped
- 1 tablespoon minced garlic
- 2 cups grated carrots
- ¼ teaspoon ground nutmeg
- ¼ cup whole-wheat pastry flour
- 2 cups low-sodium vegetable broth
- 2 cups nonfat or 1% milk
- ½ cup fat-free half-and-half
- 3 cups broccoli florets
- 2 cups shredded extra-sharp Cheddar cheese

PREPARATIONS

Using a pot, heat the olive oil over average heat and add the onion and garlic. Stir until fragrant, about 1 minute. Add the carrots and continue to stir until tender, about 2 to 3 minutes.

Add the nutmeg and the flour. Continue to cook, stirring constantly, until browned, 2 to 3 minutes. Add the broth and then the milk, and whisk constantly until it starts to thicken. Add the half-and-half and mix to combine well.

Stir in the broccoli florets. Boil and minimize to simmer. Cook for 10 minutes or until the broccoli is tender, use an immersion blender to puree it to a smooth consistency, if desired, or leave it as is for a chunky soup.

Stir in the Cheddar cheese until melted. Reserve some cheese as a topping for serving time.

Refrigerate any leftovers and eat within 1 week.

NUTRITIONAL VALUE

Per Serving (1 cup): Calories: 193; Total fat: 9g; Protein: 12g; Carbs: 17g; Fiber: 4g; Sugar: 7g; Sodium: 450mg

BARLEY-MUSHROOM RISOTTO

PREP TIME: 5 MINUTES

COOK TIME: 55 MINUTES

TOTAL TIME: 60 MINUTES

SERVINGS: 6

Barley is a nutrient-packed grain (found at a bargain price, I might add!) that you can use to replace the Arborio rice in risotto. Barley is higher in fiber, especially soluble fiber, which has been shown to lower LDL ("bad") cholesterol. I also love how this risotto dish is loaded with mushrooms and spinach to sneak in some vegetables while still maximizing flavor.

INGREDIENTS

- 1 tablespoon extra-virgin olive oil
- 1 teaspoon minced garlic
- 2 leeks, cleaned, ends removed and finely chopped, both white and green parts
- 4 cups sliced mushrooms
- 2 teaspoons dried thyme
- ½ cup pearl barley
- ½ cup dry white wine
- 1½ cups low-sodium vegetable or chicken broth
- 1 cup water
- 3 cups fresh spinach leaves

PREPARATIONS

Place a large skillet over medium heat. Sauté the olive oil and garlic for 1 minute. Add the leeks and sauté for 2 to 3 minutes, or until tender.

Add the mushrooms and cook until tender and browned, about 4 minutes.

Stir in the thyme and barley. Cook for another 2 minutes.

Add the wine and stir. Make tender for 5 minutes

Add the broth and water. Reduce the heat to low, cover the skillet, and simmer for 40 minutes. Stir occasionally to make sure the barley does not stick to the bottom of the pan.

Gently stir in the spinach and mix until it is wilted. Serve immediately.

Serving tip: Although barley is higher in protein than rice, this dish isn't particularly protein-loaded. Add some Parmigiano-Reggiano cheese, roasted tofu, or serve on the side of a chicken breast or lean pork chop to help you meet your protein goal for the day.

NUTRITIONAL VALUE

Per Serving (½ cup): Calories: 104; Total fat: 3g; Protein: 3g; Carbs: 16g; Fiber: 3g; Sugar: 1g; Sodium: 40mg

EGGPLANT ROLLATINI

PREP TIME: 15 MINUTES

COOK TIME: 50 MINUTES

TOTAL TIME: 1 HOUR, 5 MINUTES

SERVINGS: 6

Italian food is warm and comforting, yet it's often loaded with greasy beef or sausage and served with carb-laden noodles. Even vegetarian options like eggplant parmagiana still tend to be deep-fried and carb heavy. This recipe has all the flavor of a wholesome Italian dinner without the carbs and the fat. The best part is you can still eat the ooey-gooey cheese but with far fewer calories and fat than you would have with most traditional dishes.

INGREDIENTS

- Nonstick cooking spray
- 1 large eggplant
- 1 tablespoon salt
- 1 teaspoon extra-virgin olive oil
- 1 pound fresh spinach (about 10 cups)
- ½ cup part-skim ricotta cheese
- ¾ cup shredded part-skim mozzarella cheese, divided
- ¼ cup shredded Parmigiano-Reggiano cheese
- 1 egg
- 1 teaspoon minced garlic
- ½ cup Marinara Sauce with Italian Herbs or low-sugar jarred marinara sauce, divided

PREPARATIONS

Preheat the oven to 400°F. Spray 1 or 2 baking sheets with the cooking spray.

Slice the eggplant lengthwise into ¼-inch pieces. Lay the slices on a paper towel and sprinkle them with salt. Let them sit for 10 minutes to help release some of the water in the eggplant. Pat dry afterward. It's okay to wipe off some of the salt before baking.

Place the eggplant on the baking sheet and bake for 10 minutes. Remove from the oven and set aside to cool. Leave the oven on.

Put a large pot over medium-high heat. Heat the olive oil for 1 minute. Add the spinach leaves and cook, stirring occasionally, for about 3 minutes or until wilted. Set aside to let cool.

Combine the ricotta, ¼ cup of mozzarella, Parmigiano-Reggiano, egg, and garlic in a medium bowl. Mix well. When the spinach is cool, gently stir it into the cheese mixture.

Spread ¼ cup of the marinara sauce across the bottom of an 8-by-8-inch baking dish.

Spread the cheese mixture (about 2 tablespoons each) onto each eggplant slice, roll the slice, and place seam-side down in the baking dish. Continue until all eggplant slices are made into roll-ups and placed in the pan.

Top the rolled eggplant with the remaining ¼ cup of marinara and ½ cup of mozzarella.

Reduce the oven temperature to 350°F. Cover the baking sheets with aluminum foil and bake for 30 minutes. Remove the foil and bake for an additional 10 minutes, or until the cheese is brown and bubbly.

Serving tip: Pack in even more vegetables by serving over a bed of zucchini noodles or "zoodles."

NUTRITIONAL VALUE

Per Serving (2 rollatini): Calories: 160; Total fat: 7g; Protein: 11g; Carbs: 16g; Fiber: 6g; Sugar: 8g; Sodium: 330mg

CHAPTER FOUR
SIDES AND SNACKS

SIMPLE SPINACH DIP

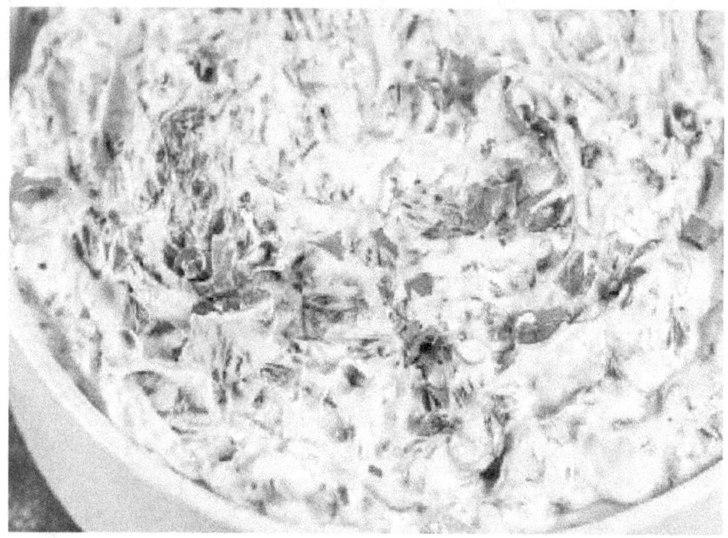

PREP TIME: 10 MINUTES
COOK TIME: 2 HOURS
TOTAL TIME: 2 HOURS, 10 MINUTES

It's certainly easy to max out on fat and calories after only a few bites of traditional spinach dip. And who can stop after only a few bites of this rich, creamy appetizer? Save on calories without compromising flavor with this simple spinach dip recipe that uses Greek yogurt instead of sour cream. Use whole seasonings and herbs instead of a premixed packet to cut back on sodium, leave out the MSG, and improve the flavor.

INGREDIENTS

- 1 cup plain nonfat Greek yogurt
- 4 ounces cheese
- ½ cup olive oil-based mayonnaise
- 2 teaspoons minced garlic
- 1½ teaspoons onion powder
- 1 teaspoon smoked paprika
- ¾ teaspoon freshly ground black pepper
- ¼ teaspoon red pepper flakes
- 2 teaspoons Worcestershire sauce
- 1 (8-ounce) can water chestnuts, drained and finely chopped
- ½ cup chopped scallions
- 1 (10-ounce) package frozen chopped spinach, thawed and squeezed of excess moisture

PREPARATION

In a large bowl, use a hand mixer on low speed to mix the yogurt, cheese, mayonnaise, garlic, onion powder, paprika, black pepper, red pepper flakes, and Worcestershire sauce.

Add the water chestnuts, scallions, and spinach and stir by hand until well combined.
Cover and refrigerate for at least 2 hours prior to serving, or overnight.
Serve with raw vegetables or whole-grain crackers.

Serving tip: Use as a spread on deli-sliced (nitrate-free) turkey and roll it up for a quick snack or a simple lunch. Or substitute for mayo or mustard on an open-face sandwich. The possibilities abound.

NUTRITIONAL VALUE
Per Serving (¼ cup): Calories: 71; Total fat: 4g; Protein: 3g; Carbs: 5g; Fiber: 1g; Sugar: 2g; Sodium: 131 mg

MASHED CAULIFLOWER

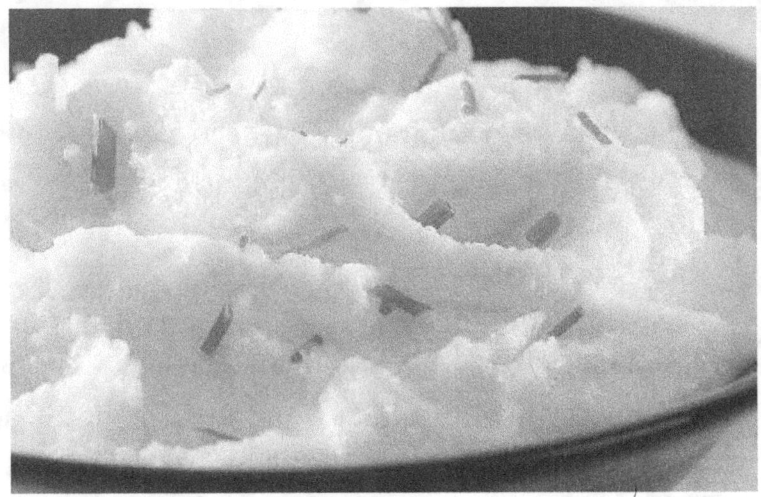

PREP TIME: 10 MINUTES
COOK TIME: 5 MINUTES
TOTAL TIME: 15 MINUTES
SERVING: 4

Potatoes are a staple of the American diet and a side dishes on many a dinner plate. Unfortunately, when we take these starchy spuds and deep-fry them or load them with butter and sour cream, we surpass our daily allowance for carbohydrates, fat, and calories. Try swapping your traditional spuds for this twist on mashed potatoes. You will save on calories and carbohydrates yet still feel comforted by the creamy nature of this simple dish.

INGREDIENTS

- 1 large head cauliflower
- ¼ cup water
- ⅓ cup low-fat buttermilk
- 1 tablespoon minced garlic
- 1 tablespoon extra-virgin olive oil

PREPARATIONS

Break the cauliflower into small florets. Place in a large microwave-safe bowl with the water. Cover and microwave for about 5 minutes, or until the cauliflower is soft. Drain the water from the bowl.

Using a food processor, puree the buttermilk, cauliflower, garlic, and olive oil on medium speed until the cauliflower is smooth and creamy.

3 Serve immediately.

Ingredient tip: You can buy buttermilk in most supermarkets, but it's just as easy to make your own. Mix 1 teaspoon freshly squeezed lemon juice with ⅓ cup low-fat milk. Let the mixture sit for about 10 minutes, or until the milk begins to thicken.

Cooking tip: For even more flavor, microwave the cauliflower with chicken or vegetable broth instead of water and add ½ cup shredded Parmigiano-Reggiano cheese when you puree the mixture. You can add protein to this dish by blending in powdered egg whites or unflavored protein powder after the first puree (puree until smooth and creamy; then add the protein powder and puree to incorporate).

NUTRITIONAL VALUE

Per Serving (½ cup): Calories: 62; Total fat: 2g; Protein: 3g; Carbs: 8g; Fiber: 3g; Sugar: 3g; Sodium: 54mg

BAKED ZUCCHINI FRIES

PREP TIME: 15 MINUTES
COOK TIME: 30 MINUTES
TOTAL TIME: 45 MINUTES
SERVINGS: 6

The salty taste of french fries is a comfort to many people—and fries are one of those foods that you can't eat just one of. After the gastric sleeve, fried food is off limits—not only because it's loaded with fat and calories, but also because it can make you feel sick. But there are plenty of healthier "fries" out there that can sate any cravings. These zucchini fries are the perfect substitute. So enjoy your next side of fries—guilt free!

INGREDIENTS

- 3 large zucchini
- 2 large eggs
- 1 cup whole-wheat bread crumbs
- ¼ cup shredded Parmigiano-Reggiano cheese
- 1 teaspoon garlic powder
- 1 teaspoon onion powder

PREPARATION

Preheat the oven to 425°F

Halve each zucchini lengthwise and continue slicing each piece into fries about ½ inch in diameter. You will have about 8 strips per zucchini.

In a small bowl, crack the eggs and beat lightly.

In a medium bowl, combine the bread crumbs, Parmigiano-Reggiano cheese, garlic powder, and onion powder.

One by one, dip each zucchini strip into the egg, then roll it in the bread crumb mixture. Place on the prepared baking sheet.

Roast for 30 minutes, stirring the fries halfway through. Zucchini fries are done when brown and crispy.

Serve immediately.

NUTRITIONAL VALUE

Per Serving (4 fries): Calories: 89; Total fat: 3g; Protein: 5g; Carbs: 10g; Fiber: 1g; Sugar: 3g; Sodium: 179mg

PICKLE ROLL-UPS

PREP TIME: 20 MINUTES
TOTAL TIME: 20 MINUTES
SERVINGS: 40

Pickles have a crisp, sour, delicious taste and almost no calories. Here is an easy recipe to make as a low-carb appetizer for your next family gathering or just for a simple snack. You can even pack them for your lunch when you're in a hurry. The pickles will satisfy your craving to "crunch" without all the added calories.

INGREDIENTS

- ¼ pound deli ham (nitrate-free), thinly sliced (about 8 slices)
- 8 ounces cheese, at room temperature
- 1 teaspoon dried dill
- 1 teaspoon onion powder
- 8 whole kosher dill pickle spears

PREPARATIONS

Get a large cutting board or clean counter space to assemble your roll-ups.

Lay the ham slices on the work surface and carefully spread on the cheese.

Season each lightly with the dill and onion powder.

Place an entire pickle on an end of the ham and carefully roll.

Slice each pickle roll-up into mini rounds about ½- to 1-inch wide.

Skew each with a toothpick for easier serving.

Did You Know? There is any number of foods with gut-healthy probiotics. Yogurt, fresh sauerkraut, and—you guessed it—pickles contain beneficial bacteria that keep your gastrointestinal tract regular and may even be linked to healthy body weight.

NUTRITIONAL VALUE

Per Serving (1 roll-up): Calories: 86; Total fat: 7g; Protein: 4g; Carbs: 4g; Fiber: 0 g; Sugar: 2g; Sodium: 540mg

TOMATO, BASIL, AND CUCUMBER SALAD

PREP TIME: 15 MINUTES

COOK TIME: 30 MINUTES

TOTAL TIME: 45 MINUTES

SERVINGS: 6

One of the most delicious parts about summertime is enjoying a refreshing salad—especially if you can make it with fresh produce from the farmers' market or your garden. The flavors and nutrients of fresh, in-season vegetables are like nothing else. This is an easy salad to make and it will complement any meal—and since it's lettuce-free, it's a great way to get out of your usual salad rut.

INGREDIENTS

- 1 large cucumber, seeded and sliced
- 4 medium tomatoes, quartered
- 1 medium red onion, thinly sliced
- ½ cup chopped fresh basil
- 3 tablespoons red wine vinegar
- 1 tablespoon extra-virgin olive oil
- ½ teaspoon Dijon mustard
- ½ teaspoon freshly ground black pepper

PREPARATIONS

In a medium bowl, mix together the cucumber, tomatoes, red onion, and basil.

In a small bowl, whisk together the vinegar, olive oil, mustard, and pepper.

Pour the dressing over the vegetables, and gently stir until well combined.
Cover and chill for at least 30 minutes prior to serving.

Serving tip: Turn this salad into a well-rounded meal by grilling up some chicken breast and cutting it into 1-inch pieces. Gently toss the chicken in the salad for a refreshing and filling lunch or dinner.

NUTRITIONAL VALUE
Per Serving (½ cup): Calories: 72; Total fat: 4g; Protein: 1g; Carbs: 8g; Fiber: 1g; Sugar: 4g; Sodium: 5mg

CHAPTER FIVE

EARLY POST-OP FOODS

VANILLA APPLE PIE PROTEIN SHAKE

PREP TIME: 5 MINUTES

TOTAL TIME: 5 MINUTES

SERVINGS: 2

Nothing feels more comfortable than fresh ice cream apple pie. This classic dessert carries warmth from the house of Mom or Grandma. Whip up this apple pie–flavored shake to taste the apple pie comfort in a drink that's low enough in calories to keep your waistline trim.

INGREDIENTS

- 1 cup of low-fat milk
- 1 scoop (1/4 cup) of vanilla protein powder
- 1 small apple, sliced, cored, and diced
- 1 teaspoon of vanilla extract
- 2 teaspoons of cinnamon ground
- 1/2 teaspoon of nutmeg
- 5 ice cubes 1 to 3 cups per day

PREPARATION

Mix the milk, protein powder, fruit, vanilla, cinnamon, musk and ice cubes in a blender. Blend for 3 to 4 minutes at high speed, until the powder is well absorbed and is no longer visible.

Bottle half the shake, and enjoy.

Refrigerate any shake that you do not instantly drink or use in an airtight container for up to 1 week. Re-blend until serving.

NUTRITIONAL VALUE

Calories: 123; total fat: 1 g; protein: 14 g; carbohydrates: 14 g; fiber: 1 g; sugar: 12 g; sodium: 153 mg;

HIGH-PROTEIN MILK MAKES

PREP TIME: 5 MINUTES

TOTAL TIME: 5 MINUTES

SERVINGS: 4

About 40 cents a cup would cost you to make and it takes in a whopping 14 grams of protein! It's a reminder that feeding into your nutrition with fancy protein powders doesn't have to be difficult. Use this recipe to make a batch for yourself to drink, use as a basis for protein shakes, or cook in milk. After a sleeve gastrectomy, this cocktail should be part of everybody's recipe box.

INGREDIENTS
- 4 cups of skim milk
- 1 cup of non-fat dry milk powder
- Post-Op Servings 1 cup, as many times a day as necessary to reach the protein goal 1 to 3 cups a day

PREPARATION

In a deep bowl or blender, slowly beat the milk and milk powder with a beater or mix at high speed for about 5 minutes until the powder is dissolved and no longer visible.

Refrigerate any of the milk you do not immediately drink or use in an airtight container. The flavour is improving instantly. After 7 days, discard any remaining milk.

NUTRITIONAL VALUE

Per Serving (1 cup): Calories: 144; total fat: 0 g; Protein 14 g; Carbs: 21 g; Fiber: 0 g; Sugar: 21 g; Sodium: 218 mg

REAL VANILLA BEAN PROBIOTIC SHAKE

PREP TIME: 5 MINUTES
TOTAL TIME: 5 MINUTES
SERVINGS: 2

Not all bacteria are produced in the same manner. Our gastrointestinal tract is loaded with bacteria which are both good and not so good. Whether our bodies are in good microbial equilibrium can impact our health. Indeed, research shows that the type of bacteria found in normal weight versus obese individuals in the intestinal tract can be different. Including foods that are rich in probiotics or healthy bacteria can help promote good overall health — particularly for the protection of the intestines. Consider this smooth, kefir-made vanilla protein shake — a fermented milk drink that is lactose-free and filled with safer bacteria than the usual yogurt cup.

INGREDIENTS

- 1 cup of unsweetened almond soy milk or low-fat milk
- 1 scoop (1/4 cup) vanilla protein powder
- 1/2 cup low-fat kefir
- 1/4 cup low-fat Greek yogurt
- 1 teaspoon vanilla extract

- 5 ice cubes 1 to 3 cups per day

PREPARATION

Mix the milk, protein powder, kefir, yogurt, vanilla and ice cubes in a blender. Mix for 3 to 4 minutes at high speed, or until the powder is well dissolved and is no longer visible.
Bottle half the shake, and enjoy.
Refrigerate any shake that you do not instantly drink or use in an airtight container for up to 1 week. Re-blend until serving.

Ingredient tip: Check for kefir in your grocery store's dairy section next to the yogurt. Mix the low-fat plain kefir into oatmeal, shakes, and smoothies overnight. Beware with sweet kefir varieties, as they are filled with lots of added sugars. To save on calories, aim for products sweetened with stevia.

NUTRITIONAL VALUE

Per Serving (1 cup): Calories: 153; Total fat: 3 g; Protein: 22 g; Carbs: 8 g; Fiber: 2 g; Sugar: 6 g; Sodium: 161 mg

PUMPKIN SPICE LATTE PROTEIN SHAKE
PREP TIME: 5 MINUTES

TOTAL TIME: 5 MINUTES

SERVINGS: 2

Imagine all packaged in one drink during the fall season. Heart-warming milk, delicious apple, spicy cinnamon, and nutmeg — this protein shake would definitely satisfy the fall craving from your favorite coffee shop for a pumpkin-spiced latte, but without all the extra sugar and fat.

INGREDIENTS

- 1 cup of low-fat milk or unsweetened soy milk
- 1/2 cup pumpkin puree
- 1 scoop (1/4 cup) vanilla protein powder
- 3/4 cup brewed decaf coffee
- 1 teaspoon ground cinnamon
- 1/4 teaspoon ground ginger
- 1/4 teaspoon ground nutmeg
- 1/8 teaspoon ground cloves 1 to 3 cups per day

PREPARATION

In a blender, add the milk, pumpkin puree, protein powder, coffee, cinnamon, ginger, nutmeg and cloves and blend well for 2 to 3 minutes, unbuttered.

Glass half the shake and enjoy.

Refrigerate any shake that you do not immediately drink or use in an airtight container for up to 1 week. Re-blend while serving.

Cooking tip: Make some spice for your own pumpkin pie. Add to smoothies, oatmeal and baked squash, or to a plain Greek yogurt flavour. Combine 2 table spoons of ground cinnamon, 1 teaspoon of ground ginger, 1 teaspoon of ground nutmeg, 1/2 teaspoon ground cloves and 1/2 teaspoon allspice ground. Keep in jar which is airtight.

NUTRITIONAL VALUE

Protein: 0 g; Carbs: 12 g; Fiber: 2 g; Sugar: 8 g; Sodium: 155 mg

PEANUT BUTTER CUP SHAKE

PREP TIME: 5 MINUTES
TOTAL TIME: 5 MINUTES
SERVINGS: 2

You may not be shocked that Reese's Peanut Butter Cups are one of the world's top-selling candies. The creamy filling of peanut butter surrounded by sweet chocolate is a treat that is difficult for most to pass over. Though after surgery, these peanut butter cups are off limits; this creamy shake will surely meet your cravings and provide plenty of protein. Use this as an afternoon snack in the office candy jar to cure your sweet tooth and to fend off grazing.

INGREDIENTS

- 1 cup of low-fat milk
- 1/2 cup of low-fat Greek yogurt
- 1/4 cup of non-fat ricotta cheese
- 1 scoop (1/4 cup) chocolate protein powder
- 2 tablespoons of peanut butter
- 2 tablespoons of cocoa powder 1 to 3 cups per day

PREPARATION

Combine the milk, yogurt, ricotta, protein powder, peanut butter powder and cocoa powder in a blender. Blend for 3 to 4 minutes at high speed, until the powders are well absorbed and are no longer visible.

Bottle half the shake, and enjoy.

Refrigerate any shake that you do not instantly drink or use in an airtight container for up to 1 week. Reblend until serving.

NUTRITIONAL VALUE

Per Serving: Calories: 215; Total Fat: 3 g; Protein: 27 g; Carbs: 18 g; Fiber: 3 g; Sugar: 11 g; Sodium: 249 mg

CHAPTER SIX
FISH AND SEAFOOD DINNERS

TUNA NOODLE-LESS CASSEROLE
PREP TIME: 15 MINUTES
COOK TIME: 40 MINUTES
TOTAL TIME: 55 MINUTES
SERVINGS: 10

Tuna noodle casserole is a classic that's quick to prepare for a weeknight meal. This noodle-less version comes to you via Matt and Diana Luttmann, who are parents of three small children. They always keep the ingredients on hand in their cupboard for a last-minute meal on those extra-busy days. This recipe is so creamy, flavorful, and delicious you won't even know the noodles are missing. The red bell pepper, tomatoes, and green beans give it just a bit of color to make it more interesting than the boring typical beige version.

INGREDIENTS

- Nonstick cooking spray
- 1 medium red onion, chopped
- 1 red bell pepper, chopped
- 1½ cups diced tomato
- 3 cups fresh green beans

- ⅓ cup olive oil-based mayonnaise
- 1 (14.5-ounce) can condensed cream of mushroom soup
- ½ cup low-fat milk
- 1 cup shredded Cheddar cheese
- ½ teaspoon freshly ground black pepper
- 8 (5-ounce) cans water-packed albacore tuna, drained

PREPARATIONS

Preheat the oven to 425°F.

Coat a large skillet with the cooking spray and place it over medium heat. Add the onion, red bell pepper, and tomatoes and sauté for about 5 minutes, or until the vegetables are tender and the tomatoes start to soften. Remove the skillet from the heat and set aside.

Cut off the stem ends of the green beans, and snap them into 3- to 4-inch pieces.

Fill a large saucepot ⅓ full with water, and place a steamer basket inside. Place the pot over high heat, and bring the water to a boil.

Add the green beans to the steamer basket, cover the pot, and reduce the heat to medium. Steam the green beans for 5 minutes. Immediately remove them from the heat, drain, and set aside.

Coat a 9-by-13-inch baking dish with the cooking spray.

In a large bowl, mix together the mayonnaise, condensed soup, milk, and cheese. Season the mixture with the black pepper.

Add the tuna, green beans, and sautéed vegetables to the bowl, and mix to combine. Pour the mixture into the baking dish.

Serve after baking for 30 minutes and brown

Cooking tip: It's easy to shake up this standby recipe. To boost protein and reduce fat, add ½ cup of nonfat cottage cheese and reduce the mayonnaise to 2 tablespoons. Use an immersion blender to puree until smooth. To change the flavor profile, first sauté the diced tomatoes in 1 teaspoon of extra-virgin olive oil for 5 minutes before cooking the rest of the vegetables.

Set the sautéed tomatoes aside and mix them in with the tuna. Then follow the rest of directions to put together the casserole. The tomatoes become almost like sun-dried and help attenuate some of the fishiness of the tuna.

NUTRITIONAL VALUE

Per Serving (1 cup): Calories: 147; Total fat: 7g; Protein: 15g; Carbs: 6g; Fiber: 2g; Sugar: 2g; Sodium: 318mg

SLOW-ROASTED PESTO SALMON

PREP TIME: 5 MINUTES
COOK TIME: 20 MINUTES
TOTAL TIME: 25 MINUTES
SERVINGS: 2

Most people in other countries consume more seafood and fish than most Americans, and not surprisingly also have lower incidence of being overweight and obese. Fish and seafood contain the same amount of protein per ounce as red meat; they're just lower in calories and saturated fat. A fellow dietitian, Michelle McDonagh, who happens to be from the beautiful country of Ireland, brought me this great salmon recipe. It's cooked slowly to help meld the flavors and keep the fish from drying out.

INGREDIENTS

- 4 (6-ounce) salmon fillets
- 1 teaspoon extra-virgin olive oil
- 4 tablespoons Perfect Basil Pesto

PREPARATIONS

Preheat the oven to 275°F. Brush the foil with the olive oil.

Place the salmon fillets skin-side down on the baking sheet.

Spread 1 tablespoon of pesto on each fillet.

Roast the salmon for about 20 minutes, or just until opaque in the center.

Serve immediately.

Cooking tip: Enjoy a gourmet meal any night of the week by keeping a bag of freshly frozen wild Alaskan salmon fillets on hand. Look for the kind that are perfectly portioned into individual fillets for easy meal prep—just thaw in the fridge a day or two before needed.

NUTRITIONAL VALUE

Per Serving (3 ounces): Calories: 182; Total fat: 10g; Protein: 20g; Carbs: 1g; Fiber: 0g; Sugar: 0g; Sodium: 90mg

HERB-CRUSTED SALMON

PREP TIME: 10 MINUTES
COOK TIME: 20 MINUTES
TOTAL TIME: 30 MINUTES
SERVINGS: 2

When it comes to power-packed protein foods, salmon is at the very top of the list. It is one of the best dietary sources of omega-3 fatty acids. Among many benefits, omega-3 fats are important for raising heart-healthy HDL cholesterol and fighting inflammation in the body. This baked salmon recipe will melt in your mouth and even non lovers of fish will delight in its tasty goodness.

INGREDIENTS

- 2 (4-ounce) salmon fillets
- 2 teaspoons minced garlic
- 1 tablespoon dried parsley
- ½ teaspoon dried thyme
- 2 teaspoons freshly squeezed lemon
- 4 tablespoons grated Parmigiano-Reggiano cheese

PREPARATIONS

Preheat the oven to 425°F. Line a rimmed baking sheet with parchment paper.

Place the salmon skin-side down on the baking sheet and cover with a second piece of parchment paper. Bake for 10 minutes.

Meanwhile, mix together the garlic, parsley, thyme, lemon juice, and Parmigiano-Reggiano cheese in a small dish.

Discard the parchment paper covering the salmon. Use a pastry brush to carefully cover the fillets with the herb-cheese mixture.

Bake the salmon, uncovered, for about 5 minutes more. The salmon is done when the fish flakes easily with a fork.

Serve immediately.

Cooking tip: Don't overcook the salmon. Overcooked fish turns rubbery and the "fishy" flavor tends to be emphasized. Fish is safely cooked when the internal temperature measures 145°F with a meat thermometer.

NUTRITIONAL VALUE

Per Serving (4 ounces): Calories: 197; Total fat: 10g; Protein: 27g; Carbs: 9g; Fiber: 1g; Sugar: 3g; Sodium: 222mg

BAKED HALIBUT WITH TOMATOES AND WHITE WINE

PREP TIME: 5 MINUTES

COOK TIME: 35 MINUTES

TOTAL TIME: 40 MINUTES

SERVINGS: 2

After the sleeve gastrectomy, many patients struggle to eat red meat as it is very dense. This halibut recipe is a great alternative to steak. While not nearly as dense as meat, it's still quite hearty. The sweetness of the Vidalia onion balanced with the tart white wine makes this dish extra delicious.

INGREDIENTS

- 3 tablespoons of extra-virgin olive oil
- 1 Vidalia onion, chopped
- 1 tablespoon minced garlic
- 1 (10-ounce) container grape tomatoes
- ¾ cup dry white wine, divided
- 3 tablespoons capers
- 1½ pounds thick-cut halibut fillet, deboned
- ½ teaspoon dried oregano
- Salt
- Freshly ground black pepper

PREPARATIONS

Preheat the oven to 350°F.

In a Dutch oven or large oven-safe skillet over medium-high heat, heat the olive oil. Add the onion and sauté until browned and softened, 3 to 5 minutes.

Add the garlic and cook until fragrant, 1 to 2 minutes.

Add the tomatoes and cook for 5 minutes, or until they start to soften. Once the tomatoes start to soften, carefully use a potato masher to gently crush the tomatoes just enough to release their juices.

Add ½ cup of the wine to the pan and stir. Cook 2 to 3 minutes until slightly thickened. Stir in the capers.

Push the vegetables to the sides of the pan leaving the center of the pan open for the fish. Place the fish in the pan and sprinkle it with the oregano, salt, and pepper, then scoop the tomato mixture over the fish.

Pour in the remaining ¼ cup of wine.

Place in the oven and bake for about 20 minutes, uncovered, or until the fish flakes easily with a fork or reaches an internal temperature of 145°F. Serve.

NUTRITIONAL VALUE

Per Serving (4 ounces): Calories: 237; Total fat: 10g; Protein: 24g; Carbs: 6g; Fiber: 1g; Sugar: 2g; Sodium: 166mg

BAKED COD WITH FENNEL AND KALAMATA OLIVES

PREP TIME: 10 MINUTES

COOK TIME: 35 MINUTES

TOTAL TIME: 45 MINUTES

SERVINGS: 4

Fennel is a vegetable commonly used in both Mediterranean and Greek cuisines that has a licorice-like flavor. Fennel is rich in the cancer-protectant antioxidant minerals magnesium and selenium, which can be in short supply after surgery.

INGREDIENTS

- 2 teaspoons extra-virgin olive oil
- 1 fennel bulb, sliced paper thin
- ¼ cup dry white wine
- ⅛ cup freshly squeezed orange juice
- 1 teaspoon freshly ground black pepper
- 4 (4-ounce) cod fillets
- 4 slices fresh orange (with rind)
- ¼ cup Kalamata olives, pitted
- 2 bay leaves

PREPARATIONS

Preheat the oven to 400°F.

Place a large Dutch oven or oven-safe skillet over medium heat and add the olive oil. Add the fennel and cook, stirring occasionally, until softened, 8 to 10 minutes.

Add the wine. Bring it to a simmer and cook for 1 to 2 minutes. Stir in the orange juice and pepper and simmer for 2 minutes more.

Remove the skillet from the heat and arrange the cod on top of the fennel mixture. Place the orange slices over the fillets. Position the olives and bay leaves around fish.

Roast for 20 minutes, or until fish is opaque. The fish is done when it flakes easily with a fork or reaches an internal temperature of 145°F. Remove the bay leaves prior to serving.

Did You Know? Olives are a great source of heart-healthy fat. Although portion control is key because they can be calorie dense, olives can bring a pop of flavor to many recipes. Try black olives on a taco salad, Kalamata olives on a Greek-themed pizza or wrap, or place a dish of mixed olives on your charcuterie board for your next dinner party.

NUTRITIONAL VALUE
Per Serving (4 ounces): Calories: 186; Total fat: 5g; Protein: 21g; Carbs: 8g; Fiber: 3g; Sugar: 4g; Sodium: 271mg

SLOW COOKER WHITE CHICKEN CHILI

PREP TIME: 10 MINUTES
COOK TIME: 6 HOURS
TOTAL TIME: 6 HOURS, 10 MINUTES
SERVINGS: 6

Hearty soups and chilis fill you up from inside out and they're great ways to pack plenty of vegetables and protein into your post-op diet. Many creamy soups are made with rich cheese or heavy cream. Try this version, which uses pureed beans to give the chili its creamy texture.

INGREDIENTS

- 2 (14.5-ounce) cans chickpeas, drained and rinsed, divided
- 2 cups low-sodium chicken broth, divided
- 1 pound boneless, skinless chicken breasts
- 1 large onion, diced
- 1 jalapeño pepper, seeded, minced
- 1 tablespoon ground cumin
- 1½ teaspoons ground coriander
- 2 teaspoons dried oregano
- 2 teaspoons chili powder
- 1 (4-ounce) can diced green chiles

- 2 cups water
- ¼ cup chopped cilantro, for garnish (optional)

PREPARATIONS

Prepare bean puree. In a blender or food processor, blend 1 can of the beans with 1 cup of broth. Set aside.

Place the chicken breasts in a 4- or 6-quart slow cooker. Top them with the onion, jalapeño, cumin, coriander, oregano, chili powder, and green chiles. Add the remaining 1 cup of broth, water, remaining 1 can of beans, and bean puree.

Cover the slow cooker, turn on low, and set the timer for 6 hours. At the 5½-hour mark, transfer the chicken to a plate and shred it with a fork. Return it to the slow cooker, and continue cooking on low for an additional 20 to 30 minutes before serving, allowing the chicken to absorb some of the liquid.

Ladle into bowls to serve and garnish with the cilantro.

Post-op tip: Eating spicy foods might help with your weight loss. When eating foods with a little extra-spicy kick, you might find you feel more satiated and eat less. The verdict is still out as to whether spicy peppers can speed your metabolism—but adding a little extra jalapeño to your chili might help you slow down and savor your meal. Bonus: Jalapeños are packed with lots of antioxidants.

NUTRITIONAL VALUE

Per Serving (1 cup): Calories: 225; Total fat: 3g; Protein: 26g; Carbs: 25g; Fiber: 7g; Sugar: 3g; Sodium: 661mg

BAKED POTATO SOUP

PREP TIME: 10 MINUTES

COOK TIME: 30 MINUTES

 TOTAL TIME: 40 MINUTES

SERVINGS: 6

Potatoes often get a bad rap for being high in carbohydrates and high in calories, but on the flip side, they are loaded with potassium and rich in fiber, among other nutrients. It's not so much the potato, but what we put on the potato that can make them less than favorable for the waistline. Soups are a fantastic way to fill up on fewer calories because the majority is liquid. Try this creamy baked potato soup. It can feed your family, or you can freeze leftovers in individual containers and use for lunches all week long.

INGREDIENTS

- 4 slices turkey bacon (nitrate-free)
- 2 tablespoons extra-virgin olive oil
- 3 tablespoons whole-wheat flour
- 1½ cups 1% milk
- 1½ cups vegetable or chicken broth
- 3 medium unpeeled russet potatoes, cut into 1-inch chunks
- ½ cup low-fat plain Greek yogurt
- ½ cup shredded sharp Cheddar cheese
- 4 tablespoons chopped chives

PREPARATIONS

Place a large stock pot over medium heat. Add the bacon and cook until crispy on both sides, turning once, about 5 minutes total. Transfer to a paper towel-lined plate to absorb any excess grease. Once cooled, chop finely and set aside.

Heat the olive oil in the stock pot over medium heat. Cook after adding flour and stir till brown for 3 minutes. Add the milk and whisk constantly until it starts to thicken. Whisk in the broth.

Add the potatoes. Boil and minimize the heat and let the soup simmer for about 20 minutes, or until the potatoes are tender.

Add the Greek yogurt and stir to combine.

Serve garnished with the turkey bacon, cheese, chives, and additional dollop of plain Greek yogurt.

Post-op tip: If you are cooking this during the post-op pureed stage, add 1 to 2 tablespoons of egg white powder or unflavored protein powder after cooking to increase the protein content.

NUTRITIONAL VALUE
Per Serving (1 cup): Calories: 181; Total fat: 9g; Protein: 9g; Carbs: 18g; Fiber: 3g; Sugar: 1g; Sodium: 174mg

CHICKEN, BARLEY, AND VEGETABLE SOUP
PREP TIME: 15 MINUTES
COOK TIME: 50 MINUTES
TOTAL TIME: 65 MINUTES
SERVINGS: 8
Think classic chicken noodle soup with a twist. Barley instead of noodles gives this soup a bit more texture and makes it more filling. The cooked vegetables are tender and easy on the stomach yet still packed with nutritious antioxidants, vitamins, and minerals. Best part: It's even better the next day as the flavors have time to meld. You can freeze this soup in small

containers to eat for lunch whenever you need a quick, warm, and filling meal.

INGREDIENTS

- 1 tablespoon extra-virgin olive oil
- 1 teaspoon minced garlic
- 1 large onion, diced
- 2 large carrots, chopped
- 3 celery stalks, chopped
- 1 (14.5-ounce) can diced tomatoes
- ¾ cup pearl barley
- 2½ cups diced cooked chicken, such as leftovers from Whole Herbed Roasted Chicken in the Slow Cooker
- 4 cups low-sodium chicken broth
- 2 cups water
- ½ teaspoon dried thyme
- ½ teaspoon dried sage
- ¼ teaspoon dried rosemary
- 2 bay leaves

PREPARATIONS

Place a large soup pot over medium-high heat. Sauté the olive oil and garlic for 1 minute.

Add the onion, carrots, and celery and sauté until tender, 3 to 5 minutes.

Add the tomatoes, barley, chicken, broth, water, thyme, sage, rosemary, and bay leaves. Bring to a simmer, then reduce the heat to medium-low and cook, uncovered, for about 45 minutes. The soup is done when the barley is tender.
Remove and discard bay leaves before serving.

NUTRITIONAL VALUE
Per Serving (1 cup): Calories: 198; Total fat: 3g; Protein: 16g; Carbs: 9g; Fiber: 2g; Sugar: 3g; Sodium: 528mg

CREAMY CHICKEN SOUP WITH CAULIFLOWER
PREP TIME: 15 MINUTES
COOK TIME: 40 MINUTES
TOTAL TIME: 55 MINUTES
SERVINGS: 8
Giving up restaurant dining and cooking more healthy meals at home doesn't mean giving up on taste and flavor. Quite the opposite. Try this knock-off version of Olive Garden's Chicken & Gnocchi Soup; it has less fat, less sodium, and fewer carbohydrates. Use leftover cooked chicken to save on meal prep time. Grill or bake several servings of chicken breast on the weekend to use

for meals throughout the week. You can even substitute canned chicken breast to save on time.

INGREDIENTS

- 1 teaspoon minced garlic
- 1 teaspoon extra-virgin olive oil
- ½ yellow onion, diced
- 1 carrot, diced
- 1 celery stalk, diced
- 1½ pounds (3 or 4 medium) cooked chicken breast, diced
- 2 cups low-sodium chicken broth
- 2 cups water
- 1 teaspoon freshly ground black pepper
- 1 teaspoon dried thyme
- 2½ cups fresh cauliflower florets
- 1 cup fresh spinach, chopped
- 2 cups nonfat or 1% milk

PREPARATIONS

Place a large soup pot over medium-high heat. Sauté the garlic in the olive oil for 1 minute
Add the onion, carrot, and celery and sauté until tender, 3 to 5 minutes.
Add the chicken breast, broth, water, black pepper, thyme, and cauliflower. Bring to a

simmer, reduce the heat to medium-low, and cook, uncovered, for 30 minutes.
Add the fresh spinach and stir until wilted, about 5 minutes.
Stir in the milk, then serve immediately.

Did You Know? Greens such as spinach, kale, and Swiss chard are all excellent sources of iron. Iron is a key nutrient for the red blood cell function of carrying oxygen to cells throughout the body. Add greens at the end of cooking soups and stews as they wilt quickly. It's a great way to use up salad greens that might be on the edge of going bad in your fridge.

NUTRITIONAL VALUE
Per Serving (1 cup): Calories: 164; Total fat: 3g; Protein: 25g; Carbs: 5g; Fiber: 1g; Sugar: 4g; Sodium: 54mg

SLOW COOKER TURKEY CHILI
PREP TIME: 10 MINUTES
COOK TIME: 8 HOURS
TOTAL TIME: 8 HOURS, 10 MINUTES
SERVINGS: 6
Chili is a simple meal to make, it has loads of flavor, and it seems to go down well post-op. Once

the chili is cooked, feel free to garnish it with plain low-fat Greek yogurt, low-fat shredded Cheddar cheese, and chopped scallions. Keep the canned ingredients in your cupboard so you can quickly toss together this meal.

INGREDIENTS

- Nonstick cooking spray
- 2 pounds extra-lean ground turkey
- 2 (14.5-ounce) cans kidney beans, drained and rinsed
- 1 (28-ounce) can diced tomatoes with green chiles
- 1 (8-ounce) can tomato puree
- 1 large onion, finely chopped
- 1 green bell pepper, finely chopped
- 2 celery stalks, finely chopped
- 4 teaspoons minced garlic
- 1 teaspoon dried oregano
- 2 tablespoons ground cumin
- 3 tablespoons chili powder
- 1 (8-ounce) can tomato juice

PREPARATIONS

Place a large skillet over medium-high heat and coat it with the cooking spray. Add the ground turkey. Using a wooden spoon, break it into smaller pieces and cook until browned, 7 to 9 minutes.

While the turkey browns, place the beans, tomatoes, tomato puree, onion, bell pepper, celery, garlic, oregano, cumin, chili powder, and tomato juice in the slow cooker. Stir in the cooked ground turkey and mix well.

Cover the slow cooker and turn on low to cook for 8 hours.

Serve garnished with Greek yogurt, shredded Cheddar cheese, and chopped scallions (if using).

NUTRITIONAL VALUE

Per Serving (½ cup): Calories: 140; Total fat: 4g; Protein: 14g; Carbs: 12g; Fiber: 4g; Sugar: 4g; Sodium: 280mg

RANCH-SEASONED CRISPY CHICKEN TENDERS

PREP TIME: 10 MINUTES

COOK TIME: 20 MINUTES

TOTAL TIME: 30 MINUTES

SERVINGS: 6

Be cautious anytime you consider eating something with the word nugget or finger in the title after chicken. More than likely you're getting a whole lot of crispy fried coating and not a lot of lean chicken breast. Skip the fast-food versions and make these chicken tenders at home. The crispy coating helps hold in all the juices to keep the chicken moist with every bite. Serve with a side of roasted vegetables or dip them in Creamy Peppercorn Ranch Dressing.

INGREDIENTS

- Nonstick cooking spray
- 6 chicken tenderloin pieces (about 1¼ pounds)
- 2 tablespoons whole-wheat pastry flour
- 1 egg, lightly beaten
- ½ cup whole-wheat bread crumbs
- 2 tablespoons grated Parmigiano-Reggiano cheese
- 2 teaspoons dried parsley
- ¾ teaspoon dried dill
- ¼ teaspoon garlic powder
- ¼ teaspoon onion powder
- ¼ teaspoon dried basil
- ⅛ teaspoon freshly ground black pepper

PREPARATIONS

Preheat the oven to 425°F.

Prepare three small dishes for coating the chicken. Place the flour in one, the egg in the second, and in the last dish mix together the bread crumbs, Parmigiano-Reggiano cheese, parsley, dill, garlic powder, onion powder, basil, and black pepper.

Working one at a time, dip each tenderloin into the flour. Shake off any excess, then dip the chicken into the egg. Finally, place the tenderloin in the bread crumbs and press to coat in the mixture. Place on the baking sheet.

Bake for about 20 minutes, or until crispy, brown and cooked through. Serve immediately.

Serving tip: Turn these into a Buffalo ranch chicken salad. Toss the crispy tenders with Frank's RedHot Buffalo Wing Sauce. Chop and place on top of a salad of mixed greens, shredded carrots, and tomatoes and top with low-fat blue cheese. Drizzle the salad with the Creamy Peppercorn Ranch Dressing.

NUTRITIONAL VALUE

Per Serving (1 chicken tender): Calories: 162; Total fat: 2g; Protein: 25g; Carbs: 8g; Fiber: 1g; Sugar: 1g; Sodium: 239mg

GRILLED CHICKEN WINGS
PREP TIME: 15 MINUTES

COOK TIME: 20 MINUTES
TOTAL TIME: 35 MINUTES
SERVINGS: 18

Whether it's for a Super Bowl party, Sunday afternoon picnic, or just a weeknight dinner—hot wings are always a fan-favorite. Most wings are breaded and deep-fried, then dredged in some sort of sugar-packed barbecue sauce. These juicy wings are grilled to perfection so the chicken falls right off the bone! Choose a buffalo wing sauce with a heat that's appropriate for you. Flaming hot sauce is optional—but go for it if that's your thing!

INGREDIENTS

- 1½ pounds frozen chicken wings
- Freshly ground black pepper
- 1 teaspoon garlic powder
- 1 cup buffalo wing sauce, such as Frank's RedHot
- 1 teaspoon extra-virgin olive oil

PREPARATIONS

Preheat the grill to 350°F.

Season the wings with the black pepper and garlic powder.

Grill the wings for 15 minutes per side. They will be browned and crispy when finished.

Toss the grilled wings in the buffalo wing sauce and olive oil.
Serve immediately.

Post-op tip: Go for the meat and skip the skin whenever possible. In the early days, weeks, and months post-op, most people will not tolerate the skin on chicken or turkey because of its dense texture. After 6 to 9 months, eating 2 or 3 deep-fried chicken wings with the skin may be tolerated, but limit portions when possible because of the high saturated fat content. Remember, everything in moderation. If wings are your favorite, you are a step ahead with this grilled version.

NUTRITIONAL VALUE
Per Serving (1 wing): Calories: 82; Total fat: 6g; Protein: 7g; Carbs: 1g; Fiber: 0g; Sugar: 0g; Sodium: 400mg

CHAPTER EIGHT
PORK AND BEEF DINNERS

CHIPOTLE SHREDDED PORK
PREP TIME: 10 MINUTES
COOK TIME: 6 HOURS
TOTAL TIME: 6 HOURS, 10 MINUTES
SERVINGS: 8

Try this slow-cooked smoky, spicy, pulled pork, which takes an otherwise tough cut of meat and makes it oh-so-tender—and thus a perfect recipe for the VSG Club. Better still, it's a simple recipe for even the most novice chef. You can toss this together on the weekend to put in the slow cooker on Monday or Tuesday for a quick weeknight meal. Serve inside low-carb taco shells for carnitas, on a low-calorie whole-wheat bun for sandwiches (try topped with a Greek yogurt–based coleslaw), or serve alongside a cup of Baked Potato Soup.

INGREDIENTS
- 1 (7.5-ounce) can chipotle peppers in adobo sauce
- 1½ tablespoons apple cider vinegar
- 1 tablespoon ground cumin

- 1 tablespoon dried oregano
- Juice of 1 lime
- 2 pounds pork shoulder, trimmed of excess fat

PREPARATIONS

Puree the chipotle peppers and adobo sauce using the blender, apple cider vinegar, cumin, oregano, and lime juice.

Place the pork shoulder in the slow cooker, and pour the sauce over it.

Cover the slow cooker, and cook on low for 6 hours.

The finished pork should shred easily. Use two forks to shred the pork in the slow cooker. If there is any additional sauce, allow the pork to cook on low for 20 minutes more to absorb the remaining liquid.

Post-op tip: Variety is the spice of life, but is it the best method for weight loss? Sometimes having similar types of meals on a daily basis, such as the same breakfast or lunch, can help limit the guesswork and keep calories or portions controlled. Although it's important to get a variety of nutrients in your diet—it's A-OK to use a simple meal plan to keep yourself on track!

NUTRITIONAL VALUE

Per Serving (½ cup pork): Calories: 260; Total fat: 11g; Protein: 20g; Carbs: 5g; Fiber: 2g; Sugar: 2g; Sodium: 705mg

ONE-PAN PORK CHOPS WITH APPLES AND RED ONION

PREP TIME: 10 MINUTES
COOK TIME: 30 MINUTES
TOTAL TIME: 40 MINUTES
SERVING: 4

These pork chops are flavorful and melt-in-your-mouth tender. The sweet cooked apples are a perfect balance for the savory pork—that's why it's a classic combination. Plus, you can keep a clean kitchen by using just one pot. Try serving with Roasted Root Vegetables as a side dish or over Cauliflower Rice.

INGREDIENTS

- 2 teaspoons extra-virgin olive oil, divided
- 4 boneless center-cut thin pork chops
- 2 small apples, thinly sliced
- 1 small red onion, thinly sliced
- 1 cup low-sodium chicken broth

- 1 teaspoon Dijon mustard
- 1 teaspoon dried sage
- 1 teaspoon dried thyme

PREPARATIONS

Place a large nonstick frying pan over high heat and add 1 teaspoon of olive oil. When the oil is hot, add the pork chops and reduce the heat to medium. Sear the chops for 3 minutes on one side, flip, and sear the other side for 3 minutes, 6 minutes total. Put the chops by the side

In the same pan, add the remaining 1 teaspoon of olive oil. Add the apples and onion. Cook for 5 minutes or until tender, stirring frequently to prevent burning.
While the apples and onion cook, mix together the broth and Dijon mustard in a small bowl.

Add the sage and thyme to the pan and stir to coat the onion and apples. Stir in the broth mixture and return the pork chops to the pan. Cover the pan and simmer for 10 to 15 minutes.
Let pork chops rest for 2 minutes before cutting.

NUTRITIONAL VALUE

Per Serving (1 pork chop): Calories: 234; Total fat: 11g; Protein: 20g; Carbs: 13g; Fiber: 3g; Sugar: 9g; Sodium: 290mg

SLOW COOKER PORK WITH RED PEPPERS AND PINEAPPLE

PREP TIME: 10 MINUTES

COOK TIME: 5 HOURS

TOTAL TIME: 5 HOURS, 10 MINUTES

SERVINGS: 4

Depending on how it's prepared, pork can be a tough meat. With a smaller stomach after the sleeve gastrectomy, you might have a harder time digesting dense foods. This slow-cooked pork is naturally tenderized by the enzymes in the pineapple. I recommend using canned pineapple since it seems to be less fibrous than fresh. Serve the pork by itself or over Cauliflower Rice. This meal freezes well and stays moist when reheated.

INGREDIENTS

- ¼ cup low-sodium soy sauce or Bragg Liquid Aminos
- Juice of ½ lemon
- 1 teaspoon garlic powder
- 1 teaspoon ground cumin
- ½ teaspoon cayenne pepper

- ¼ teaspoon ground coriander
- 1½ pounds boneless pork tenderloin
- 2 red bell peppers, thinly sliced
- 2 (20-ounce) cans pineapple chunks in 100% natural juice or water, drained

PREPARATIONS

In a small bowl, mix together the soy sauce, lemon juice, garlic powder, cumin, cayenne pepper, and coriander.

Place the pork tenderloin in the slow cooker and add the red bell pepper slices. Cover with the pineapple chunks and their juices. Pour the soy sauce mixture on top.

Cover the slow cooker and turn on low for about 5 hours.

Shred the pork with a fork and tongs and continue to cook on low for 20 minutes more, or until juices are absorbed.

Serve and enjoy!

Ingredient tip: If you're not familiar with Bragg Liquid Aminos, it is a liquid protein concentrate, derived from soybeans. It contains all 16 amino acids and has a taste that's very similar to soy sauce.

NUTRITIONAL VALUE

Per Serving (3 ounces): Calories: 131; Total fat: 2g; Protein: 17g; Carbs: 11g; Fiber: 2g; Sugar: 8g; Sodium: 431mg

PORK, WHITE BEAN, AND SPINACH SOUP
PREP TIME: 10 MINUTES
COOK TIME: 40 MINUTES
TOTAL TIME: 50 MINUTES
SERVINGS: 6

Pork and beans just seem to go well together. This soup pairs the rich, smoky flavor of pork with savory spinach and white beans. It's a simple recipe to toss together on a weeknight. Sear the pork before making the rest of the soup to lock in the juices and to keep the meat tender.

INGREDIENTS

- 1 teaspoon extra-virgin olive oil
- 1 medium onion, chopped
- 2 (4-ounce) boneless pork chops, cut into 1-inch cubes
- 1 (14.5 ounce) can diced tomatoes
- 3 cups low-sodium chicken broth
- ½ teaspoon dried thyme
- ¼ teaspoon crushed red pepper flakes

- 1 (15-ounce) can great northern beans, drained and rinsed
- 8 ounces fresh spinach leaves

PREPARATIONS

Place a large soup pot or Dutch oven over medium heat and heat the olive oil.

Add the onion and sauté for 2 to 3 minutes, or until tender. Add the pork and brown it for 4 to 5 minutes on each side.

Mix in the tomatoes, broth, thyme, red pepper flakes, and beans. Boil and minimize heat to simmer, covered, for 30 minutes.

Add the spinach and stir until wilted, about 5 minutes, and serve immediately.

Did You Know? Pork (and all meats, eggs, and dairy) is an excellent source of vitamin B12, which is important for preventing anemia and is crucial for nerve function. Because of changes in the absorption of vitamin B12 and a risk of its deficiency after bariatric surgery, many patients need a B12 supplement in the form of a pill or injection. Eating foods that are high in vitamin B12 is a good way to keep those levels topped up.

NUTRITIONAL VALUE

Per Serving (1 cup): Calories: 156; Total fat: 4g; Protein: 17g; Carbs: 17g; Fiber: 4g; Sugar: 6g; Sodium: 600mg

SPAGHETTI SQUASH CASSEROLE WITH GROUND BEEF

PREP TIME: 10 MINUTES

COOK TIME: 75 MINUTES

TOTAL TIME: 1 HOUR, 25 MINUTES

Nothing like a dish of spaghetti with beef sauce to fill an empty stomach after a long day of work

Just because you can't have starchy pasta doesn't mean you can't have a meal just as comforting, with cheese and beef and only one-third of the carbs. Prepare to be satisfied with loads of cheese and beefy goodness as you swap pasta for spaghetti squash in this casserole recipe.

INGREDIENTS

- Nonstick cooking spray
- 2 medium spaghetti squash (2½ to 3 pounds)
- 1 pound supreme lean ground beef
- 1 large onion, minced
- 2 teaspoons minced garlic
- 1 (8-ounce) can tomato sauce

- 1 (10-ounce) can diced tomatoes
- 1 teaspoon dried basil
- 1 teaspoon dried oregano
- 1 cup shredded mozzarella cheese
- ½ cup shredded Parmigiano-Reggiano cheese

PREPARATIONS

Preheat the oven to 350°F. Coat a baking sheet with the cooking spray.

Halve the spaghetti squash, remove and discard the stem, pulp, and seeds, and place the halves cut-side down on the baking sheet. Bake till the flesh is tender and for 35 minutes.

While the squash bakes, spray a large skillet with the cooking spray, and place it over medium heat. Add the ground beef, onion, and garlic, and sauté for about 10 minutes, or until the beef is no longer pink and the onion is tender. Add the tomato sauce, diced tomatoes, basil, and oregano and stir to combine well. Remove the pan from the heat and set aside.

When the spaghetti squash is cool enough to handle, carefully use a fork to pull the flesh from the outer skin and make "spaghetti." Set aside in a bowl.

In a 9-by-13-inch baking dish, layer one-third of the meat-and-tomato mixture in the bottom of the dish. Evenly spread half of the squash over the meat layer. Layer another one-third of the meat mixture over the squash. Finish the last layer with the second half of the squash and the last one-third of the meat mixture. Sprinkle the mozzarella and Parmigiano-Reggiano cheeses over the top. Cover with aluminum foil and bake for 30 minutes. Remove the foil and bake for 10 minutes more, or until the cheese begins to brown. Serve.

Cooking tip: Going vegetarian? Replace the beef in this recipe with ground soybeans or another vegetarian ground beef alternative. Add an additional ½ cup water to the "meat"-and-tomato mixture to keep it moist.

NUTRITIONAL VALUE

Per Serving (1 cup): Calories: 229; Total fat: 10g; Protein: 20g; Carbs: 16g; Fiber: 3g; Sugar: 11g; Sodium: 511mg

CREAMY BEEF STROGANOFF WITH MUSHROOMS

PREP TIME: 10 MINUTES
COOK TIME: 30 MINUTES

TOTAL TIME: 40 MINUTES
SERVIMGS: 6

There's nothing more filling than wholesome beef Stroganoff to fill you up when you're feeling hungry, but the combination of high-fat creamy sauce and rich beef in traditional recipes won't agree with your sleeve after surgery. Try this healthier twist on the traditional recipe made with simple staple ingredients from your kitchen. Serve over zucchini noodles or Cauliflower Rice instead of pasta to keep carbohydrate servings in check.

INGREDIENTS

- Nonstick cooking spray
- 1½ pounds extra-lean beef sirloin, cut into ½-inch strips
- 1 teaspoon extra-virgin olive oil
- 1 medium onion, chopped
- ½ pound mushrooms, sliced
- 2 tablespoon whole-wheat flour
- 1 cup low-sodium beef broth
- 1 cup water
- 1 teaspoon Worcestershire sauce
- ½ teaspoon dried thyme
- ½ teaspoon dried dill
- ½ cup low-fat plain Greek yogurt

- 2 tablespoons finely chopped fresh parsley, for garnish

PREPARATIONS

Coat a medium pan with the cooking spray and place over medium-high heat. Add the beef. Cook, stirring frequently, until browned, about 5 minutes. Transfer to a bowl and set aside.

In the same pan, heat the olive oil over medium-high heat. Add the onion and cook until tender, 1 to 2 minutes.

Add the mushrooms and cook until tender, about 3 minutes.

Mix in the flour and stir to coat the onion and mushrooms.

Stir in the broth, water, Worcestershire sauce, thyme, dill. Bring to a boil, cover the pan, and cook for about 10 minutes, stirring frequently.

Stir in the yogurt. Mix in the beef. Serve, garnished with the parsley.

NUTRITIONAL VALUE

Per Serving (4 ounces): Calories: 351; Total fat: 9g; Protein: 31g; Carbs: 30g; Fiber: 5g; Sugar: 5g; Sodium: 418mg

ITALIAN BEEF SANDWICHES

PREP TIME: 10 MINUTES

COOK TIME: 7 HOURS

TOTAL TIME: 7 HOURS, 10 MINUTES

SERVINGS: 6

Before weight-loss surgery you may have enjoyed the occasional beef sandwich laden with sauce and served on a doughy bun. This is a fantastic recipe for a slow-cooked beef sandwich, but with a healthy twist. Using a slow cooker to prepare beef helps get the perfect texture for when you add more red meat back to your diet.

INGREDIENTS

- 1 cup water
- 1 tablespoon balsamic vinegar
- ¾ teaspoon garlic powder
- ¾ teaspoon onion powder
- 1½ teaspoons dried parsley
- ¾ teaspoon dried oregano
- ¼ teaspoon dried thyme
- ½ teaspoon dried basil
- ¼ teaspoon freshly ground black pepper

- 1½ pounds boneless beef chuck roast, fat trimmed
- 1 medium onion, sliced
- 1 red bell pepper, cut into strips
- 6 sprouted-grain hot dog buns or sandwich thins
- 1 (16-ounce) jar pepperoncini (optional)

PREPARATIONS

In a small bowl mix together the water, balsamic vinegar, garlic powder, onion powder, parsley, oregano, thyme, basil, and black pepper.

Place the beef in the slow cooker and add the onion and bell pepper.

Pour the sauce over the roast. Cover the slow cooker and cook on low for 7 hours. The meat should be tender and cooked through.

Carefully transfer the roast to a cutting board.

Thinly slice the roast.

Toast the buns or sandwich thins.

Layer each bun with the beef and top with the au jus, pepper, and onion. Serve with pepperoncini (if using).

Post-op tip: A word about starches: Doughy bread products are not well tolerated after weight-loss surgery and should be avoided to help keep carbohydrate counts down. Most people find that eventually they can tolerate toasted bread products—but the thinner, the better (no large deli rolls). For this recipe you may decide to forgo the bun altogether and serve up the meat with vegetables, or you may try just half of a bun. Always focus on eating protein first before filling up on carbohydrates.

NUTRITIONAL VALUE
Per Serving (1 sandwich): Calories: 351; Total fat: 9g; Protein: 31g; Carbs: 30g; Fiber: 5g; Sugar: 5g; Sodium: 418mg

CHAPTER NINE
SWEETS AND TREATS

CHOCOLATE BROWNIES WITH ALMOND BUTTER

PREP TIME: 5 MINUTES
COOK TIME: 25 MINUTES
TOTAL TIME: 30 MINUTES
SERVINGS: 16

Make cocoa powder a pantry staple. It will give you the chocolate flavor without all the fat, sugar, and calories of traditional milk chocolate. These chocolate brownies have all the fudgy texture of a boxed mix but are made with healthy fat and agave nectar. Although agave is a sugar, it has a lower glycemic index than white sugar and may raise the blood sugar more gradually. If you don't like almond butter, feel free to replace it with smooth peanut butter.

INGREDIENTS

- Nonstick cooking spray
- ½ cup cocoa powder
- 1 tablespoon ground flaxseed
- ½ teaspoon ground instant coffee
- ¼ teaspoon baking soda

- ½ cup almond butter
- ¼ cup melted coconut oil
- 2 large eggs
- 1 teaspoon vanilla extract
- ½ cup agave nectar

PREPARATIONS

Preheat the oven to 325°F. Coat an 8-by-8-inch glass baking dish with the cooking spray.

Place the cocoa powder, flaxseed, instant coffee, baking soda, almond butter, coconut oil, eggs, vanilla, and agave nectar in a high-speed blender or food processor. Blend on medium-high until smooth. Pour the batter into the baking dish.

Bake for 25 minutes or until a toothpick inserted in the middle comes out clean. Let cool for 10 minutes before cutting into 16 squares.

Serving tip: Allowing dessert but concerned about overdoing the servings? Portion out the brownies and freeze them in freezer-safe resealable bags or containers. Thaw one serving at a time to allow yourself an occasional treat.

NUTRITIONAL VALUE

Per Serving (1 brownie): Calories: 124; Total fat: 9g; Protein: 3g; Carbs: 11g; Fiber: 2g; Sugar: 9g; Sodium: 49mg

EASY PEANUT BUTTER COOKIES

PREP TIME: 15 MINUTES
COOK TIME: 15 MINUTES
TOTAL TIME: 30 MINUTES
SERVINGS: 15

Sometimes you need a sweet treat and you don't have a lot of time to mix together a long list of ingredients. These easy four-ingredient peanut butter cookies are low in sugar since they're made with stevia, but so tasty they will certainly satisfy your sweet tooth.

INGREDIENTS

- Nonstick cooking spray
- 1 cup natural smooth peanut butter
- 1 large egg
- ½ cup stevia baking blend
- ½ teaspoon vanilla extract

PREPARATIONS

Preheat the oven to 350°F. Coat a nonstick baking sheet with the cooking spray or use parchment paper.

In a medium bowl, use a hand mixer to combine the peanut butter, egg, stevia, and vanilla.

Roll the batter into 1-inch balls and place them on the baking sheet. Flatten each ball to about ¼-inch thickness. Using a fork, create two imprints of a crisscross pattern on the cookie.

Bake for about 12 minutes. The cookies are done when golden brown.

Cool for 5 minutes, then move to a baking rack to finish cooling.

Ingredient tip: Peanut butter is dense in calories and fat—but it's loaded with good-for-you and heart-healthy monounsaturated fat. Choose natural versions that require you to mix the oil and peanut paste together. Stay away from any versions that include partially hydrogenated oils (trans fats) or palm oil (saturated fat). Many commercial versions in which the peanuts and oil are already mixed together also contain added sugars. Stick to the cleaner version and enjoy in moderate portions to keep calories in check.

NUTRITIONAL VALUE

Per Serving (1 cookie): Calories: 107; Total fat: 9g; Protein: 4g; Carbs: 4g; Fiber: 1g; Sugar: 2g; Sodium: 47mg

LEMON-BLACKBERRY FROZEN YOGURT

PREP TIME: 10 MINUTES

TOTAL TIME: 10 MINUTES

SERVINGS: 10

Cool and creamy ice cream and frozen yogurt go hand in hand with the hot days of summer. While your previous iced favorites might be off limits after weight-loss surgery, this frozen yogurt will satisfy your urge for ice cream. It takes just four ingredients and can be made in less than 10 minutes, which means you can enjoy this dessert all summer long.

- **INGREDIENTS**
- 4 cups frozen blackberries
- ½ cup low-fat plain Greek yogurt
- Juice of 1 lemon
- 2 teaspoons liquid stevia
- Fresh mint leaves, for garnish

PREPARATIONS

In a blender or food processor, add the blackberries, yogurt, lemon juice, and stevia. Blend until smooth, about 5 minutes.

Serve immediately or freeze in an airtight container and use within 3 weeks. Garnish with fresh mint leaves.

Serving tip: Get creative and mix and match unique flavors for your fro-yo. Use flavored Greek yogurt (low-sugar versions, if possible) as a base, and mix and match other fruits and herbs to switch it up! Try watermelon with lime and cayenne pepper or coconut with mango.

NUTRITIONAL VALUE

Per Serving (⅔ cup): Calories: 68; Total fat: 0g; Protein: 3g; Total Carb: 15g; Fiber: 5g; Sugar: 11g; Sodium: 12mg

NON-BAKED PEANUT BUTTER PROTEIN BITES WITH DARK CHOCOLATE

PREP TIME: 20 MINUTES

COOK TIME: 30MNIUTES

TOTAL TIME: 50 MINUTES

SERVINGS: 25

Energy bites, superfood balls, power squares . . . these little nutrient-packed snacks can be found lining the shelves of your health food and grocery stores for a high price. Make them at home for less money and an even better taste. These protein bites are packed with energy in the form of nutrient-dense ingredients and calories, so portion control is an absolute must. But with a great combination of carbohydrates, fat, and protein, they are an excellent pre- or post-workout snack—bring them along for your next hiking adventure!

INGREDIENTS

- 1 cup old-fashioned rolled oats
- 1 cup vanilla protein powder
- ¾ cup smooth natural peanut butter
- 2 tablespoons ground flaxseed
- 1 tablespoon chia seeds
- 1 teaspoon vanilla extract
- ¼ cup dark chocolate chips
- ¾ teaspoon stevia baking blend
- 1 tablespoon water (or more or less to reach desired consistency)

PREPARATIONS

Mix together the oats, protein powder, peanut butter, flaxseed, chia seeds, vanilla, chocolate chips, stevia, and water in a large mixing bowl.

Refrigerate for at least 30 minutes.

Roll into 25 balls and Store in a refrigerator after being packaged in an airtight sheet.

Eat within 1 week or freeze.

Cooking tip: Mix and match the dry or wet ingredients to make simple swaps. Add coconut and cocoa powder for a chocolate fix, or try sunflower seed butter instead of peanut butter to go nut-free. You can also add some pumpkin puree and cinnamon for a fall treat.

NUTRITIONAL VALUE

Per Serving (2 bites): Calories: 181; Total fat: 10g; Protein: 11g; Carbs: 11g; Fiber: 3g; Sugar: 3g; Sodium: 105mg

LOW-CARB CRUSTLESS CHERRY CHEESECAKE

PREP TIME: 10 MINUTES

COOK TIME: 45 MINUTES, PLUS 2 HOURS TO CHILL

TOTAL TIME: LESS THAN 3 HOURS

SERVINGS: 25

I'm always on the lookout for great, crowd-pleasing desserts that don't have all the added sugar and fat. I hit the jackpot with this creamy cheesecake recipe. It's a melt-in-your-mouth cheesecake topped with sweet and tart cherries. Enjoy this recipe guilt-free after surgery.

INGREDIENTS

FOR THE CHEESECAKE

- Nonstick cooking spray
- 2 (8-ounce) packages Neufchâtel cheese, at room temperature
- Juice of ½ lemon
- ¼ cup nonfat plain Greek yogurt
- 2 teaspoons vanilla extract
- ¼ cup stevia baking blend
- 3 large eggs

For the topping

- 12 ounces frozen cherries, stemmed and pitted
- 2 tablespoons water
- 2 teaspoons cornstarch
- 1 teaspoon stevia baking blend

PREPARATIONS

TO MAKE THE CHEESECAKE

Preheat the oven to 325°F. Coat a 9-inch springform pan or pie plate with the cooking spray.

In a large bowl, mix together the cheese, lemon juice, yogurt, and vanilla.

Add the stevia and mix until smooth.

Next mix in the eggs, one at a time, until well blended, Pour the filling into the pan.

Bake till the center is set for approximate 45 minutes. When done, the cheesecake should be slightly browned and barely firm in center.

TO MAKE THE TOPPING

While the cheesecake bakes, place a medium pot over medium-high heat. Put the cherries and water in the pot and bring to a boil, then reduce the heat to medium-low. Simmer until the cherries begin to bubble.

Stir 2 tablespoons of the cherry juices into the cornstarch. Stir this slurry into the cherries. This will thicken the topping. Stir in the stevia. Remove the pot from the heat and set aside to cool.

Cool the cheesecake for 30 minutes before refrigerating. Refrigerate for at least 2 hours, or overnight, before serving.

Serve with the cherry topping.

NUTRITIONAL VALUE

Per Serving (1 piece with cherry topping): Calories: 156; Total fat: 10g; Protein: 6g; Carbs: 7g; Fiber: 1g; Sugar: 5g; Sodium: 215mg

CHAPTER TEN
DRESSINGS, SAUCES, AND SEASONINGS

GREEK SALAD DRESSING
PREP TIME: 10 MINUTES
TOTAL TIME: 10 MINUTES
SERVINGS: 1

When people are trying to lose weight, a lot of effort is put into eating salads. I always get questions about salad dressing. Do I get diet? Or regular? Creamy? Oil-based? Here's the verdict: Diet dressings contain fewer calories, but they are often packed with added sugars and sodium. Oil- and vinegar-based dressings are heart healthy but can still be calorie dense so portions should be limited. There are a lot of options for creamy salad dressings made with yogurt that are suitable replacements for the traditional creamy dressings that are higher in fat. The best dressing? The one you make at home. You can control the ingredients and the flavor is out of this world! The added bonus is you won't ever have to waste time scrutinizing labels in the dressing aisle again.

INGREDIENTS
- ⅓ cup extra-virgin olive oil

- Juice of 1 lemon
- 4 teaspoons minced garlic
- 1 tablespoon dried oregano
- 1 teaspoon dried basil
- ½ teaspoon freshly ground black pepper
- ½ teaspoon Dijon mustard
- ½ cup red wine vinegar

PREPARATIONS

In a medium bowl, whisk together the olive oil, lemon juice, garlic, oregano, basil, pepper, and mustard. Alternatively, place these ingredients in a dressing shaker bottle and shake until combined.

Whisk in the red wine vinegar until emulsified.

Serve immediately. Refrigerate any leftovers in an airtight container. When ready to use, let the dressing sit for 10 to 15 minute at room temperature prior to serving in case the oil has solidified. Give it a whisk or a shake before dressing your salad.

Serving tip: Make salad exciting again by swapping your traditional iceberg lettuce salad for a Mediterranean-inspired Greek salad. Add flavorful dressing to romaine lettuce, sliced red onion, Kalamata olives, pepperoncini, feta cheese, and grilled chicken.

NUTRITIONAL VALUE

Per Serving (2 tablespoons): Calories: 89; Total fat: 9g; Protein: 0g; Carbs: 1g; Fiber: 0g; Sugar: 0g; Sodium: 3mg

SEAFOOD SAUCE

PREP TIME: 10 MINUTES
TOTAL TIME: 10 MINUTES
SERVINGS: 2

We already know that boiled or baked seafood is one of the lowest-calorie ways to eat protein, plus you get all those brain- and heart-healthy omega-3s. But you don't have to eat them plain. Adding a little seafood sauce, rich with flavor from fresh lemon and horseradish, can take your seafood from boring to a zesty party in your mouth.

INGREDIENTS

- 1½ cups catsup (free of high-fructose corn syrup)
- 2 tablespoons grated horseradish
- Juice of 1 lemon
- 1 tablespoon Worcestershire sauce

- 1 teaspoon chili powder
- ¼ teaspoon freshly ground black pepper

PREPARATIONS

In a small bowl, combine the catsup, horseradish, lemon juice, Worcestershire sauce, chili powder, and pepper. Refrigerate, covered, for at least 30 minutes or overnight to let the flavors meld.

Serve with shrimp cocktail, oysters, grilled scallops, or other seafood.

Post-op tip: Use this as a base to enjoy your favorite seafood selections on the pureed diet.

NUTRITIONAL VALUE

Per Serving (¼ cup): Calories: 56; Total fat: 0g; Protein: 0g; Carbs: 14g; Fiber: 0g; Sugar: 10g; Sodium: 445mg

CREAMY PEPPERCORN RANCH DRESSING

PREP TIME: 10 MINUTES

TOTAL TIME: 10 MINUTES

SERVINGS: 1

For many people ranch dressing is one they can't live without. It not just the most commonly used salad dressing on veggies, but it's also good on burgers, as a dip for almost anything, and as a sandwich spread instead of mayo. The problem with most ranch dressings is that they are loaded with fat, salt, artificial additives, and preservatives. Swap the mayo and heavy cream for Greek yogurt and add natural spices and herbs, toss in a blender, and voilà!—you have a delicious homemade creamy dressing that is the perfect topping for all your favorites.

INGREDIENTS

- ¾ cup low-fat plain Greek yogurt
- ⅓ cup grated Parmigiano-Reggiano cheese
- ¼ cup low-fat buttermilk (see here for tip to make from scratch)
- Juice of 1 lemon
- 2 teaspoons freshly ground black pepper
- ½ teaspoon onion flakes
- ¼ teaspoon salt

PREPARATIONS

Using a blender puree the yogurt, cheese, buttermilk, lemon juice, pepper, onion flakes, and salt on medium-high speed until the dressing is completely smooth and creamy.

Serving tip: This ranch dressing is great as a dip for raw vegetables, a condiment for a turkey wrap with vegetables, or a topping for your next turkey burger.

NUTRITIONAL VALUE
Per Serving (2 tablespoons): Calories: 35; Total fat: 1g; Protein: 4g; Carbs: 2g; Fiber: 0g; Sugar: 1g; Sodium: 133mg

HOMEMADE ENCHILADA SAUCE
PREP TIME: 5 MINUTES
COOK TIME: 10 MINUTES
TOTAL TIME: 15 MINUTES
SERVINGS: 2

Does this sound familiar? You have all the ingredients to make enchiladas, but you have no sauce. No need to run to the grocery store at the last minute when you can whip up this quick version from simple pantry staples. Mixing all the herbs and seasonings together in a fresh batch makes this sauce super tasty without any added sodium or other artificial ingredients. You might never waste your money on the canned version again!

INGREDIENTS
- 2 tablespoons extra-virgin olive oil
- ¼ cup chopped onion

- 1 teaspoon minced garlic
- 2 tablespoons whole-wheat pastry flour
- 1 tablespoon chili powder
- ½ teaspoon dried oregano
- ½ teaspoon smoked paprika
- 1 teaspoon ground cumin
- 1 cup low-sodium vegetable or chicken broth
- ½ cup water
- 1 medium tomato, seeded and chopped

PREPARATIONS

Place a small saucepan on the stove over medium heat. Add the oil, onion, and garlic. Sauté for 1 to 2 minutes, or until tender

Add the flour. Continue stirring until the onion and garlic are evenly coated.

Mix in the chili powder, oregano, paprika, and cumin. Gradually whisk in the broth and water, whisking constantly to prevent lumps from forming.

Add the tomato. Cook for 8 to 10 minutes, stirring frequently, or until mixture has thickened, Use an immersion blender to puree the tomato chunks until smooth. Alternatively, transfer the sauce to a blender and puree until smooth.

Serve immediately. You can also freeze and use at a later date.

NUTRITIONAL VALUE

Per Serving (2 tablespoons): Calories: 37; Total fat: 0g; Protein: 0g; Carbs: 7g; Fiber: 2g; Sugar: 4g; Sodium: 17mg

PERFECT BASIL PESTO

PREP TIME: 5 MINUTES
TOTAL TIME: 5 MINUTES
SERVINGS: 5

Pesto isn't just for pasta. It's also an easy-to-make flavorful spread for meat and burgers, or a tasty topping for zoodles. Remember to think of pesto as a fat, not a sauce. You need to use only a very small amount to get loads of flavor in your food. Divide it into mini containers and freeze. Then you just need to thaw one small portion at a time.

INGREDIENTS

1 cup fresh basil leaves
¼ cup Parmigiano-Reggiano cheese
2½ tablespoons extra-virgin olive oil
2 tablespoons pine nuts
2 tablespoons water

PREPARATIONS

Place the basil, Parmigiano-Reggiano, olive oil, pine nuts, and water in a food processor or blender. Pulse until smooth
Serve immediately or keep in an airtight container before serving.

Ingredient tip: Pine nuts can be pricey. You may substitute an equal portion of walnuts or almonds as a quick and inexpensive replacement for pine nuts.

NUTRITIONAL VALUE

Per Serving (1 tablespoon): Calories: 99; Total fat: 10g; Protein: 2g; Carbs: 1g; Fiber: 0g; Sugar: 0g; Sodium: 68mg